THIS BOOK

BELONGS TO

....

....

Thank you for Purchasing my book and taking the time to read it from front to back. I am always grateful when a reader chooses my work and I hope you enjoyed it!

With the vast selection available online, I am touched that you chose to be purchasing my work and take valuable time out of your life to read it. My hope is that you feel you made the right decision.

I very much would like to know what you thought of the book. Please take the time to write an honest and informative review on Amazon.com. Your experience and opinions will be of great benefit to me and those readers looking to make an informed choice.

With much thanks.

Chapter 1: Overview

Chapter 2: Why It Is Essential to Workout When You Are a New Mother

Chapter 3: Readiness Check- When And How To Start Exercising After Delivery

    How to Start Exercising After Delivery

Chapter 4. Best Home Workouts for New Mothers!

Chapter 6: Nutrition While Breastfeeding and Exercising

Conclusion

Chapter 1: Overview

The female body changes immensely during pregnancy and continues changing even after delivery. These changes and transformations are necessary to accommodate the baby and its needs.

During pregnancy, the additional weight comes from the baby, the placenta, amniotic fluid, and the breast tissues increase in preparation for nursing the baby, the growing uterus, and a store of fats used to make milk after the baby's birth.

After the baby's birth, your weight reduces because the baby is no longer in your uterus, with the placenta expelled, and your body does not have to retain as much fluid. However, your body still retains fat reserves, a lot of fluids are added in the course of labor and delivery, and the body holds on to that for a week after that. You will be able to notice a difference in your weight after about three weeks after shedding the extra fluids retained during labor.

In general, women gain 13.5Kgs to 18Kgs during pregnancy (or more), depending on each person's situation. After the baby is born, about 10 Kgs to 13 Kgs of this weight comes out with the baby in the first three weeks. Whether you lose weight after this or not mainly depends on how much you eat, your food choices, and your activity levels.

While you may be very enthusiastic about losing the baby weight as soon as possible, it is best to focus on healing and establishing your milk supply. After that, you can then start working on your nutrition and working out.

We will cover more on nutrition in a later chapter. Right now, we will focus on working out and how beneficial it is to work out when you are a new mother.

The next chapter will focus on the benefits of exercising as a new mother and why home workouts are your best bet as a new mom.

Chapter 2: Why It Is Essential to Workout When You Are a New Mother

When you become a mother, you may find that time becomes somehow limited because you will spend most of it taking care of the little one or working. Resultantly, you may lack time to work out.

Many women shy away from working out because they feel like they have to exercise at the gym or away from home. However, plenty of exercises are light, safe, and doable at home. The good thing about this is that you only need just a few minutes every day or at least regularly; say sparing around 15-30 minutes every day to work out, and a month will be enough to notice the difference.

How do you stand to benefit by working out?

Aside from helping you lose the baby weight and regain your body shape, exercise offers other crucial benefits to you as a new mom. Below are the key benefits of working out as a new mum.

Exercise is an energy booster

Taking care of a newborn is a lot of work, and many mothers complain of being low on energy. However, did you know that working out can boost your energy levels? Each time you work out, you build your endurance. The higher your endurance, the more you can engage in several activities without feeling like you are getting tired quickly, which is a plus considering how demanding taking care of a baby can be.

It improves your mood and prevents postpartum depression

Working out improves your physical and mental health. People who exercise are generally happier than people who don't because exercising increases the endorphin levels circulating in your body.

Endorphins are chemicals the body produces when we indulge in pleasurable activities such as sex and a good laugh. When you exercise, the body produces more endorphins, leaving you feeling good —endorphins are what cause the "runners high."

It helps you sleep better

Exercise helps you get high-quality, longer sleep. When you work out, you tire the muscles, and they need time to recover. The recovery happens during your sleep. When you engage in physical activity, by the end of the day, you are ready to have some rest. When you wake up, you feel fresh and energized because your muscles recovered during sleep

It helps you lose extra weight and regain your ideal weight

When you exercise and watch what's on your plate, you will eventually have a calorie deficit that will lead to weight loss.

NOTE: You will still need to be aware of the calories you consume daily because you still need enough to produce adequate milk for the baby.

It helps strengthen and tone abdominal muscles

Pregnancy stretches your abdominal muscles to give way for the uterus to grow. This separates the abdominal muscles into two, a condition called Diastasis Recti. After giving birth, the muscles get back together during healing. Exercise can help you heal the muscles, strengthen them, and tone your abdomen.

It is important to note that abdominal workouts after childbirth should be done very carefully and only if you're physically ready to strain your abdomen.

It is best to consult your doctor before doing these exercises, especially if you delivered your baby through a caesarian section; you could easily damage the wound if you start exercising pre-maturely.

With that understanding of the importance of working out as a new mother, I believe you would want to know when is the best time to start working out.

Let us find out in the next chapter.

Chapter 3: Readiness Check- When And How To Start Exercising After Delivery

Your birth experience will determine how soon you can begin exercising. Whether you had any complications is something you cannot ignore.

It is okay to do light exercises like Kegel exercises and short walks after vaginal and caesarian section births within the first week of having your baby.

Moderate to light exercises are recommended after six weeks for mothers who had a vaginal birth with no complications. Doctors feel that your body has healed at six weeks and can take light exercises. However, this is very general, and it is best to listen to your body and consult your doctor to confirm if it is safe to start exercising.

Doctors recommend exercising eight to three months of delivery for mothers who have their babies through caesarian births. However, this recommendation is general and depends on individual situations and birth experiences. The birth scar needs time to heal completely. Exerting unnecessary pressure on the wound/scar could damage the tissues around it and cause more pain and problems for the mother. Consult your gynecologist to clear you for any form of exercise after a cesarean birth.

How to Start Exercising After Delivery

Pregnancy separates the six-pack muscle into two from the linea alba fiber —see the image below.

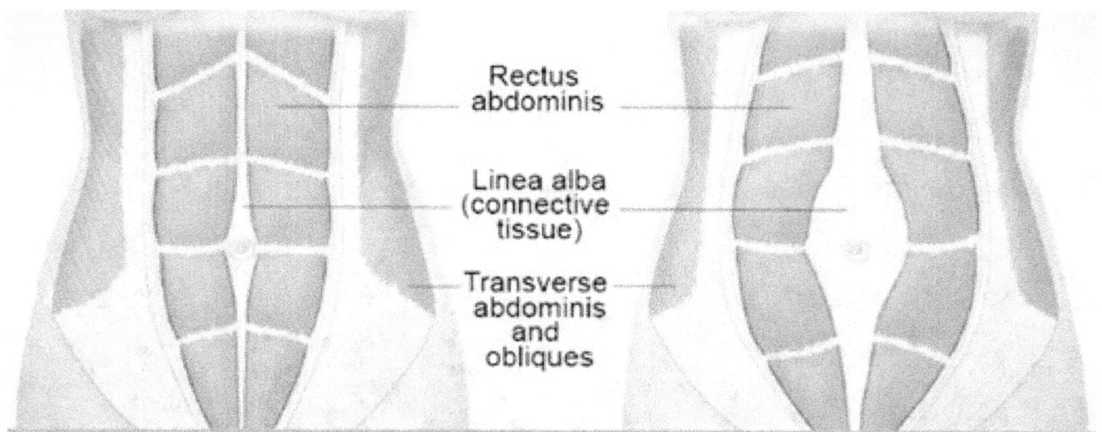

After delivery, these muscles should get back together at the linea alba once again –we called this separation condition Diastasis Recti. It is what causes the stomach to bulge for months after delivery. We do a self-check called a Rec check to check if the six-pack muscles have healed and reconnected.

To do the Rec check, lie down on a mat with your back against the mat, knees raised, and feet on the ground. Using two or three fingers, begin to feel the six-pack muscles to tell how big the separation is.

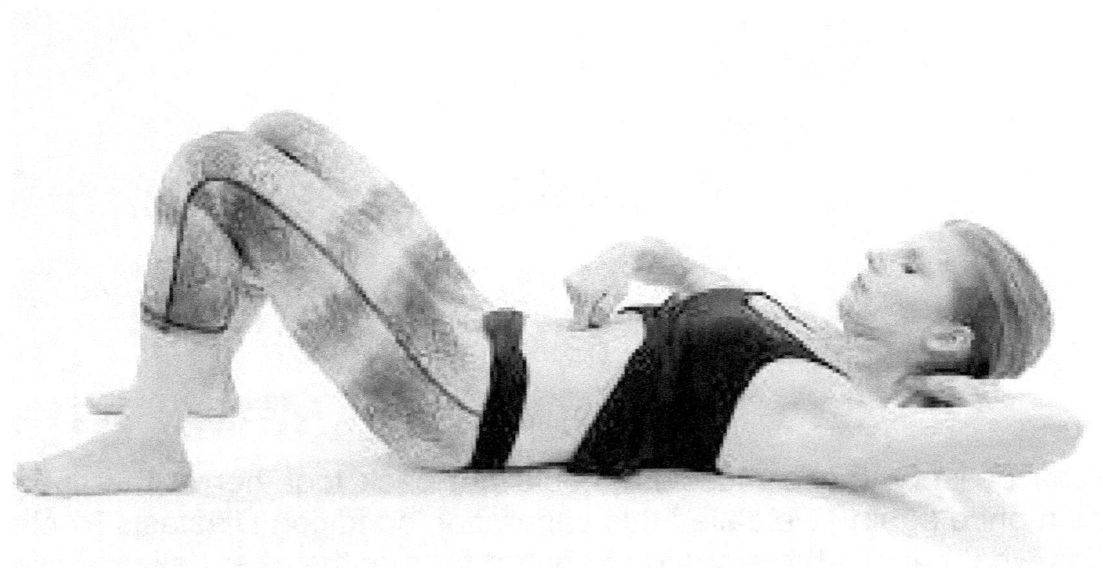

While in the same position, with your fingers on your abdomen, lift your head slightly so that your hand can feel the squeeze of your muscles. You want to use your fingers to determine if the six-pack muscles are separate. If your muscles have healed, you should not feel the separation.

With one-two finger space between your muscles, you can do simple exercises such as Pilates. When done properly, Pilates can help you seal the separation because such exercises exert pressure on the spine and towards the linea alba.

Exercises that push out the abdomen are not suitable for you at this point.

This is the test exercise; to confirm the kind of exercises your body can handle. For a visual illustration of how to do this exercise, check out the YouTube video below:

https://www.youtube.com/watch?v=uAZZNssjbVE

Do not ignore warning signs such as bleeding, vaginal/abdominal pain, discomfort in your pelvic area, and urine or body fluids leakage.

Before working out every time, ensure you hydrate to keep your joints well-lubricated.

You will also need to take time to warm up. Warming up helps you pay attention to your body and detect any pain. If you feel pain, stop exercising because it shows you haven't healed completely.

Another vital thing to remember is to wear a supportive bra with nursing pads in case breast milk starts leaking during exercise.

The next chapter gives detailed effective workouts you can do as a new mom.

Chapter 4. Best Home Workouts for New Mothers!

To make this chapter easier to navigate and read, we have classified the workouts based on the body part they target.

You can decide to have a schedule to exercise particular parts on particular days, full-body on some other days, or even combine the workouts as per your preference.

These workout categories include:

1. Cardio workouts
2. Belly / Abdominal workouts
3. Lower body/ Leg workouts
4. Upper body workouts

Cardio Workouts

Cardio exercises aim to raise your heart rate, which causes the heart to pump blood faster, causing higher oxygen circulation, which keeps your heart and lungs healthy.

The cardio workouts in this book are subdivided into beginner, intermediate, and advanced cardio workouts.

The beginner and intermediate cardio workouts are light and safe, while the advanced cardio workouts are ideal for when you feel confident in your stability and strength level.

Beginner and Intermediate level Cardio Workouts

These include:

#: *Walking*

Starter exercises should be low impact. Walking is the most recommended exercise after child delivery. It is safe to walk after a week of having a baby, depending on your unique situation. You can start with a stroll, and it doesn't even have to be outside your home. You can walk around your home. You could also alter your walking style by walking backward or in a zigzag to ensure you can feel the impact on several muscles.

You can walk for around 15-30 minutes every day to see results.

#: *Jogging in place*

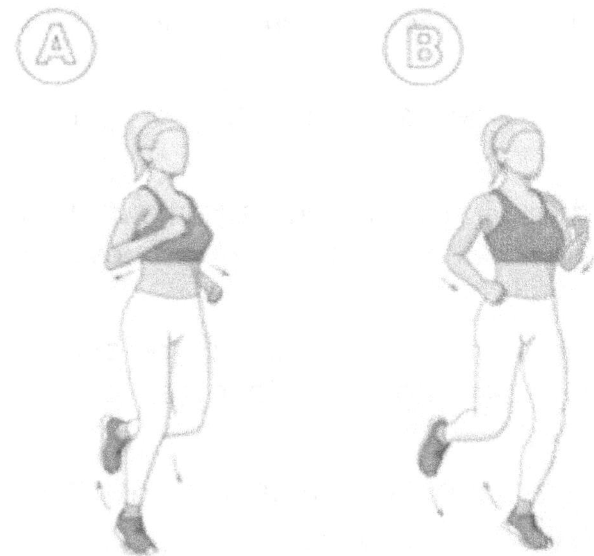

Jogging in place involves running in one spot without moving forward or backward.

How to jog in place

- Lift the right leg at the same time as the right arm. The arm goes just at chest level or slightly above the chest.
- Bring your right foot and arm down.

- Lift your left leg immediately and quickly, using the same style as the right leg and arm.

- Bring the left foot back to the ground,

- Continue with the same movements,

- Start at a slow pace and increase the pace slowly.

- Do this at intervals of 4 minutes, then take a rest of two minutes.

If this is uncomfortable for you, you can do its modified version, which does not require you to jump, but lift your legs slowly, one after the other consistently, without stopping. You can do it at a pace that is comfortable for you.

The benefits of jogging are the same as running but not as intense, which is okay.

You are also not limited to jogging in place. You can take it further to jogging in circles around the house or outside, whatever feels comfortable for you.

This exercise puts pressure on your hips and ankles; you should not continue if you feel pain, you can move on to other low-impact exercises or give it a rest.

Jogging in place and walking have the same impact on the body, but walking is easier on your body than jogging in place.

But in essence, they both improve cardio health, build strength, and burn calories.

#: Modified Jumping Jacks

Jumping jacks is a total body workout you can do comfortably at home.

Jumping jacks strengthen your muscles, from hamstrings to glutes, hips, calves, shins, and quads; they also work your heart and lungs.

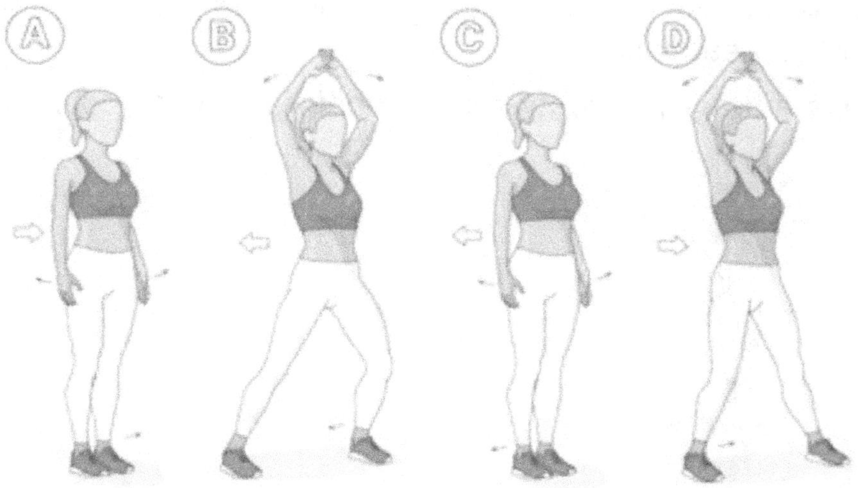

<u>How to do modified jumping jacks:</u>

- The normal jumping jacks involve jumping up while moving both legs from the middle to having them apart and bringing them back together in the middle every time you jump.

- Simultaneously lift your arms as if waving both of them. They should meet above your head.

- Repeat this movement quickly at a comfortable pace.

With modified jumping jacks, instead of jumping:

- You move your arms the same way as if you're waving with both to meet above your head.

- Then move each leg at a time from middle to sideways and back to the middle.

- Repeat these movements at your own pace but don't stop for thirty seconds

- Take a break of twenty seconds before you can continue.

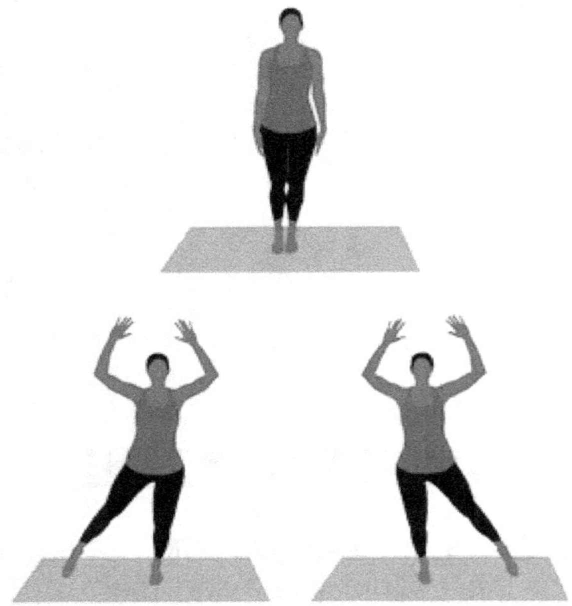

Another modification of the jumping jack is where you:

- Lift your right arm above your head towards the left, then bring it down to the waist level.

- Move your right leg outwards or sideways while also moving your right arm and back to the middle.

- Lift your left arm immediately, the same way, above the head towards the right, and bring it down towards the waist.

- Move the left foot outside to the side, simultaneously with the left arm, then bring it back to the middle.

- Continue with these movements for thirty seconds.

Your speed depends on your comfort level but ensure you do not stop until the thirty seconds are over so that you will feel the impact of the jumping jacks.

Stop if you feel pain and try out other friendlier workouts.

Jumping jacks generally, if done correctly, should not be harmful to you. It is best to do jumping jacks on a flat surface like grass ground, but the floor on your house is also fine, provided it is flat.

You should do jumping jacks two to three days a week, especially during the first weeks of starting workouts postpartum.

#: Modified Fast Feet and Punch

Fast punches are interesting workouts that make you move your feet very fast while at the same time coordinating with fast punches to race your heart and work on your hamstrings.

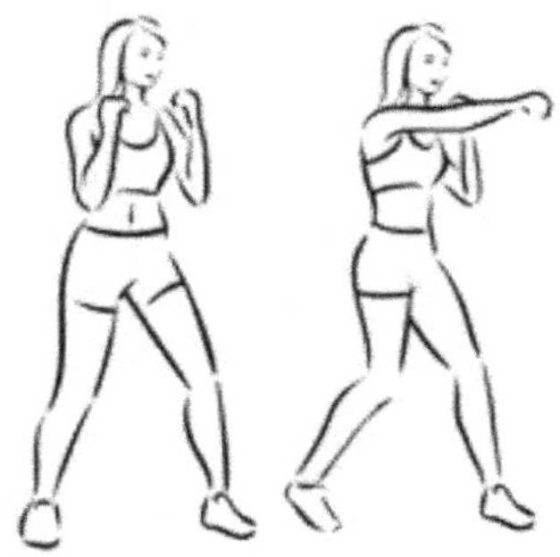

- First, start by standing straight with feet slightly apart.

- Bend your knees slightly and have your back straight and spine neutral.

- Bend your arms and have your fists under your chin.

- Begin to take fast, shuffling, and alternating steps.

- As you take the steps, extend your arms to make quick alternating punches; you should be throwing quick, short punches and making quick, shuffling steps with your feet.

- Do this for 30 seconds without stopping. Take a ten minutes break and do two more sets.

Advanced Cardio Workouts

These include:

#: Jumping rope

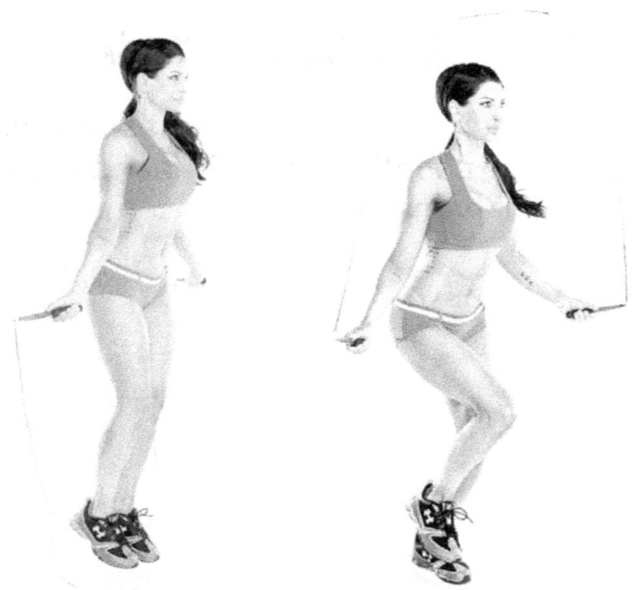

Jumping rope is another exercise that gets your heart racing, improving blood circulation and muscle strength.

Jumping rope may not be suitable before six weeks of birth. After six or eight weeks, when you feel your body is ready, you can jump rope as a cardio exercise after clearance from your doctor.

<u>How to jump rope</u>

- Place your elbows close to your body while holding the rope in both hands, then jump and continue jumping while swinging the rope from below your feet to above your head and repeat these movements.

- Start at a slow pace and a few jumps each day. The slow pace helps you assess your body and determine if the exercise agrees with your body.

- Land softly on your toe tips when you jump, and do not jump too high; jump gently at low heights but continuously so that your heart feels the impact.

- When you are comfortable jumping, you can try out other tricks with the rope.

- Jump rope twenty to twenty-five minutes after every two days, and later, you can jump every day.

#: Modified Burpees

Burpees are higher intensity than jumping jacks and jumping rope. They're whole-body workouts that involve continuous squats, pushups, and jumps. Burpees work to strengthen the shoulder, arms, chest, abdomen, hips, legs, and glute muscles. They're those workouts that you feel are difficult before you even start but leave you dripping sweat, refreshed, and feeling good.

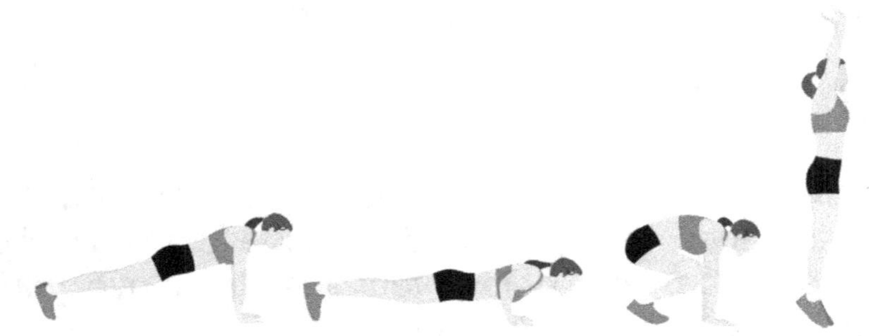

However, if you are not comfortable with the regular burpees, you can modify them to make them easier but still effective cardio workouts.

<u>The normal burpees involve:</u>

- While standing straight on your feet, go into a squat position, with your hands touching the ground.
- Kick your feet back so that now you're in a pushup position.
- Do one pushup and then immediately go back into a squat position.
- From the squat position, jump and clap or tap your palms together above your head.
- Repeat the moves without stopping.

That is the normal intense burpee. You can modify this to eliminate the jump, which may be uncomfortable, or eliminate the pushup. Let's look at the first modification without jumping.

- To start, be in an upright standing position.
- Bend and touch the ground or your feet with your hands.

- While bending and with your hands touching the ground, begin walking backward with your feet. Walk as further as possible to put you in a position ready for a pushup.

- Do one pushup, then return to the pushup-ready position.

- From the pushup position, begin walking forward with your feet only, to the bending position, with your hands still on the ground.

- Now stand upright and clap your hands above your head.

- Repeat these moves twenty times without stopping.

Only stop if you feel pain; otherwise, push yourself to complete the workout.

The other variation of burpees eliminates the pushups. So you will be in a pushup position, but instead of doing the pushup, you will start walking back to the bent position, before standing up into an upright position and clapping your hands above your head.

You can also modify the pushup to have your knee on the ground so that instead of doing it from your feet, you do it from your knees like below.

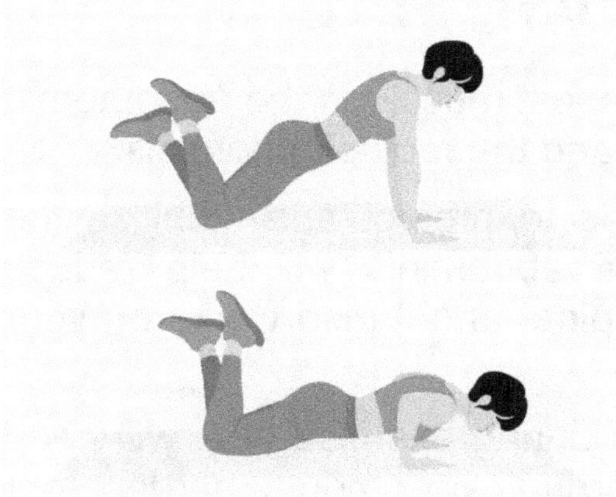

Belly/Abdominal Workouts

Belly workouts are popularly called core abdominal or Abs workouts.

It is normal to have sagging skin around your belly after weeks, months, or even a year after delivery. Most belly workouts will help you tone up the belly area.

There are many options for abdominal workouts and core workouts that can help you repair diastasis recti and strengthen the tummy muscles while burning the extra fat accumulated around the belly area.

Let's first take a moment to understand the abdominal muscles and to know the names given to these muscles.

#: *The Rectus Abdominis Muscle*

The rectus abdominis is a muscle that extends from the pubic bone to the rib cage and is divided in the middle by a verticle fibrous line called the linea alba and horizontally by tendinous intersections to form a 'six-pack.'

The rectus abdominis muscle is easily seen and felt in people with low body fat.

Transversus abdominis

The transversus abdominis is the deepest muscle in the abdomen; it sits below the rib cage, the obliques, and the rectus abdominis.

The transverse abdominis function is to protect and stabilize the spine. Strengthening the transverse abdominis will help reduce lower back pain by stabilizing your spine, and it also works on your waistline

To engage the transverse abdominis during exercise, you will need to draw your belly in and exhale air through your mouth, harden your pelvic and belly muscles, and begin breathing normally with your belly still held in.

Once you have mastered engaging your inner abdominal muscles, you will feel and see the effects of your workouts with time.

Internal and external obliques

The internal and external obliques are the muscles found on the side of the abdomen; in other words, they are the lateral abdominal walls that make part of the waist muscles.

The external oblique runs from the rib down to the hips, while the internal obliques are deeper muscles found below the external obliques and run from the ribs to the pubic bone.

The oblique muscles give flexion and rotation to the abdominal trunk. They also give tension to the abdominal wall, which is important during childbirth, breathing, and urination for all humans; it also supports the internal organs.

The oblique muscles connect to the rectus abdominis –that is why they're all part of the core. When you exercise your rectus abdominis, it also indirectly exercises the obliques.

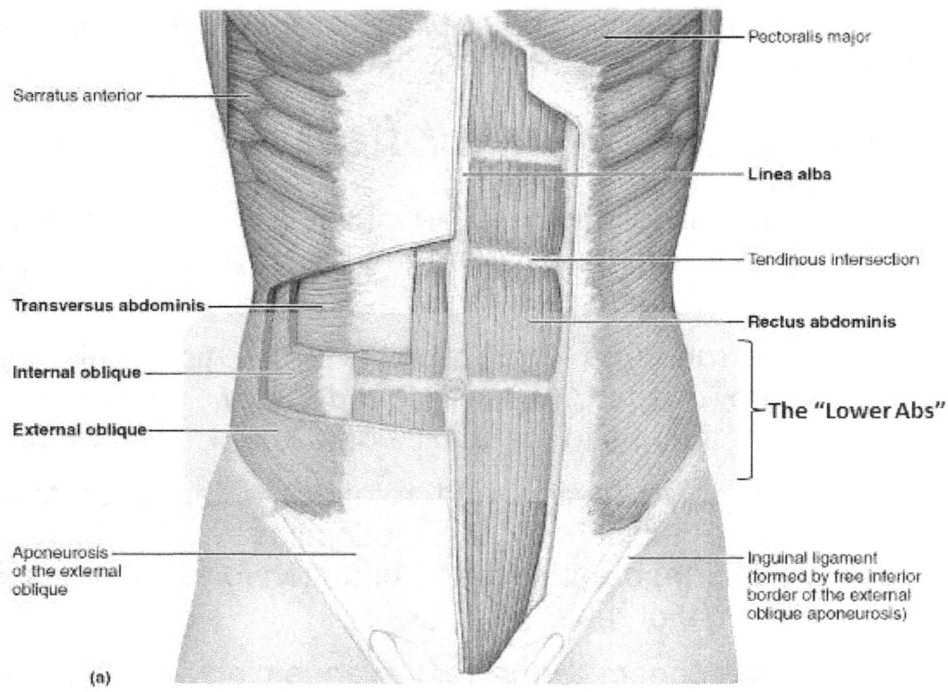

Doing abdominal exercises incorrectly can lead to an abdominal hernia, while exercising the core correctly can heal an abdominal hernia. That makes it important to understand these muscles and their functions.

We will break our abdominal exercises into three.

1. Beginner, light abdominal exercises

2. Intermediate abdominal exercises and

3. High-intensity abdominal exercises.

This subdivision will help you try out exercises at your level.

Beginner Light Abdominal Exercises

These include:

Pelvic tilts

Because they are one of those exercises that work on your pelvic muscles while also strengthening the abdominal muscles, Pelvic tilts will be your base exercise, especially when working to heal diastasis recti.

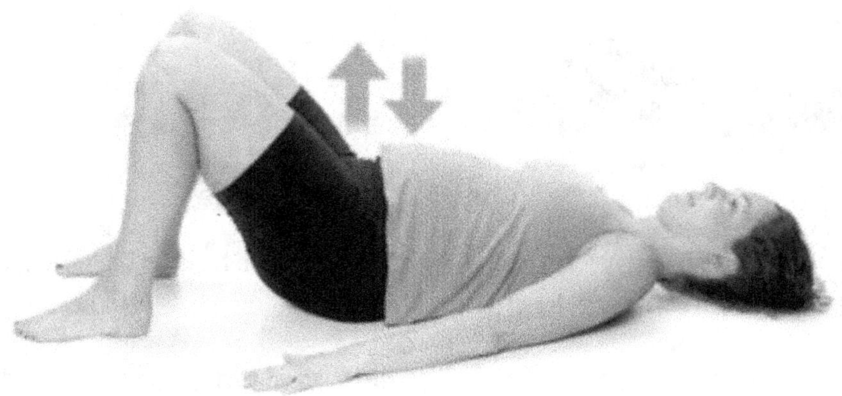

- Lie on your back on flat ground, with your knees bent. Move your feet as close as possible to your butt.

- Relax in that position, then draw your belly button towards your spine. Your spine should be flat against the floor. Remain that way, with your belly button drawn in for ten seconds, then relax.

- Repeat these movements twenty times without stopping.

You can also do the pelvic tilt while standing.

- Ensure your back is straight and your knees slightly bent.
- Engage your abdominal muscles by drawing your belly button towards your spine, just like you did lying on your back, then repeat the exercise for at least ten minutes.

#: Heel slide-outs

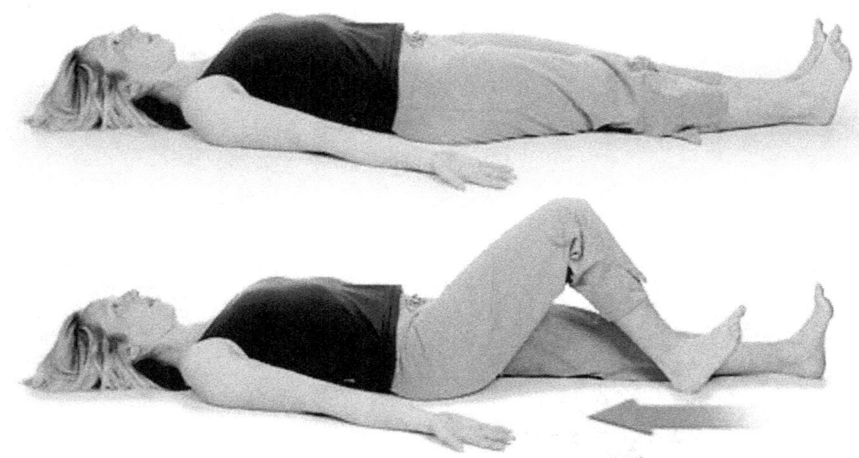

Since you now know how to do the pelvic twist, the heel slides will be an additional move to the pelvic twist.

- Lie on the ground, flat like you did when we did the pelvic tilts, with your knees bent and feet flat on the ground.
- Engage your abdominal muscles, then slide one heel until your leg is straightened up.
- Lift the same leg back in knee bent position.
- Do this with the other heel.
- Repeat these moves twenty times.

You can modify the heel slide-outs to have your legs stretched out straight against the ground instead of having your knees bent.

Then slide your heel upwards towards your butt and back into the flat position.

Do this for both heels and repeat twenty times.

#: Lying leg raises

There are two ways to do the lying leg raises. You can lift both legs or lift one leg at a time.

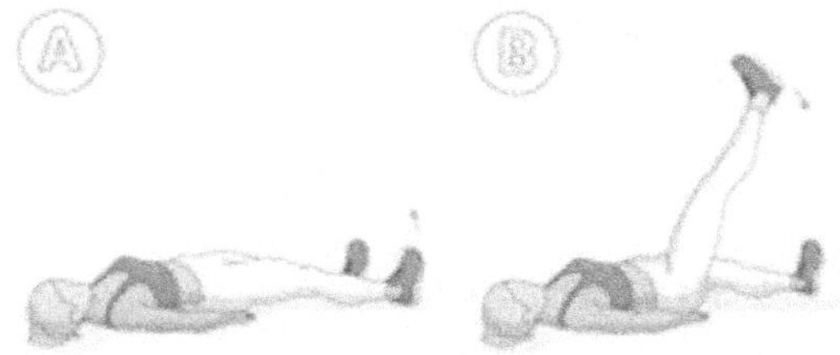

- Lie flat on the ground with your feet straight against the floor.

- Your hands should extend straight against the ground –as shown in the image above.

- Engage your abdominal muscles by hardening them.

- Raise one leg to a 45-degree angle, then return it to the ground.

- Slowly lift the other leg to a 45-degree angle and return it to the ground.

- Repeat ten times, take a ten-second break, then do another ten lifts.

The other way to do this exercise is to lift both legs simultaneously to the 45-degree angle, just as we have done with the single-leg raises.

#: Alternating knee hug

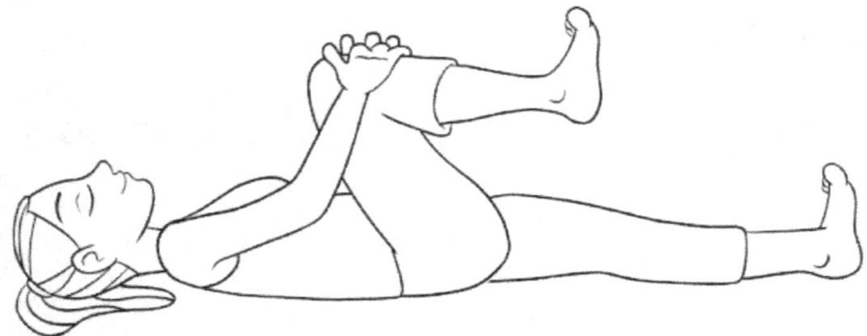

- Lie on the ground with legs straight.

- Engage your abdominal muscles by drawing them inwards. This strengthens the abdominal muscles and works towards bringing them back together.

A situation where the muscles bulge to form a cone is discouraged because it will create even a deeper separation that we are working to seal.

- Lift one knee to hug it on your chest, then return the leg to the starting position.

- Switch to the other knee and hug it against your chest and return it to the starting position

- Repeat ten times for each leg.

You can intensify the knee hugs by not returning your feet to the ground after the hug; instead, keep it raised off the ground.

#: Standing bicycle crunches

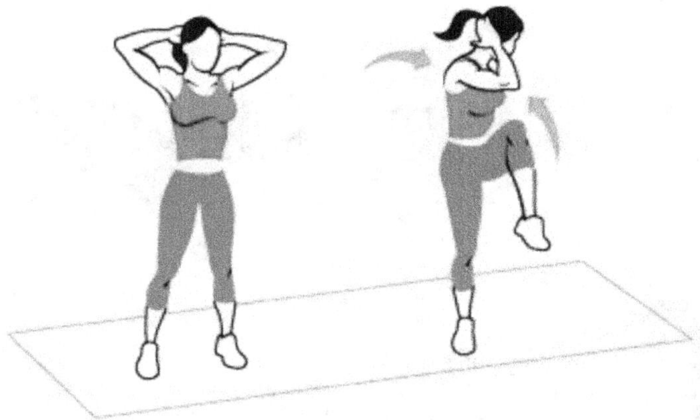

Standing bicycle crunches exercise the abdomen:

- Stand straight on flat ground, with your feet apart
- Place both hands at the back of your head
- Lift your knee to touch your opposite knee with your opposite elbow.
- Do the same with the other knee with its opposite elbow.
- Do this while drawing your abdomen inwards
- Repeat ten times for each side.

You can modify the standing bicycle to make it easier. Instead of having your hands at the back of your head, have your arm folded to touch the knee with the elbow. Repeat ten times for each side.

#: Alternating toe taps

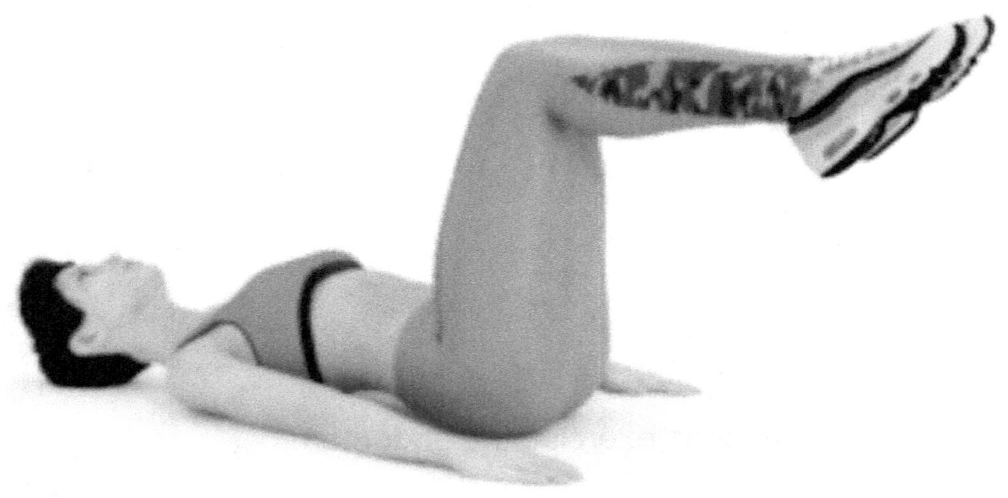

- Lie on your back on flat ground, with your hands flat on the ground as well

- Lift your legs and bend the knees; keep them in that position.

- Engage your abdominal muscles by drawing your abdomen inside.

- Tap the ground with the toe of one leg and immediately return the leg to its bent position.

- Tap the ground with the other leg and return it to the bent knee position.

- Repeat the same moves alternating the legs ten times for each leg.

#: Wall pushups

When done right, wall pushups engage your upper body, the back, and abdominal muscles.

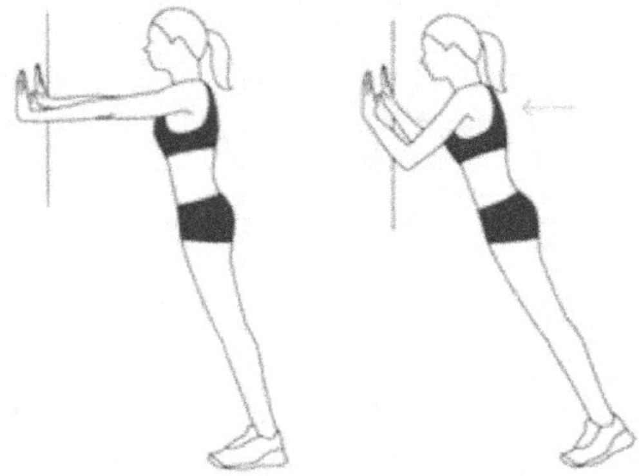

- Stand arms' length away from the wall, facing the wall, feet slightly apart, and legs straight.

- Place your hands on the wall, slightly wider than shoulder length.

- Push your body towards the wall, closest to the wall but don't touch the wall

- Immediately push yourself back to an arms-length distance away from the wall

- Repeat this twenty times.

Intermediate Abdominal Exercise

The intermediate abdominal exercises are more intense than the beginner abdominal exercises. You can do these once your abdominal muscles have built up some stamina and when you are feeling more comfortable engaging the abdominal muscles.

These exercises include:

#: Glute Bridges

As the name suggests, glute bridges work your glutes but are also a great exercise to strengthen your core and hamstring muscles.

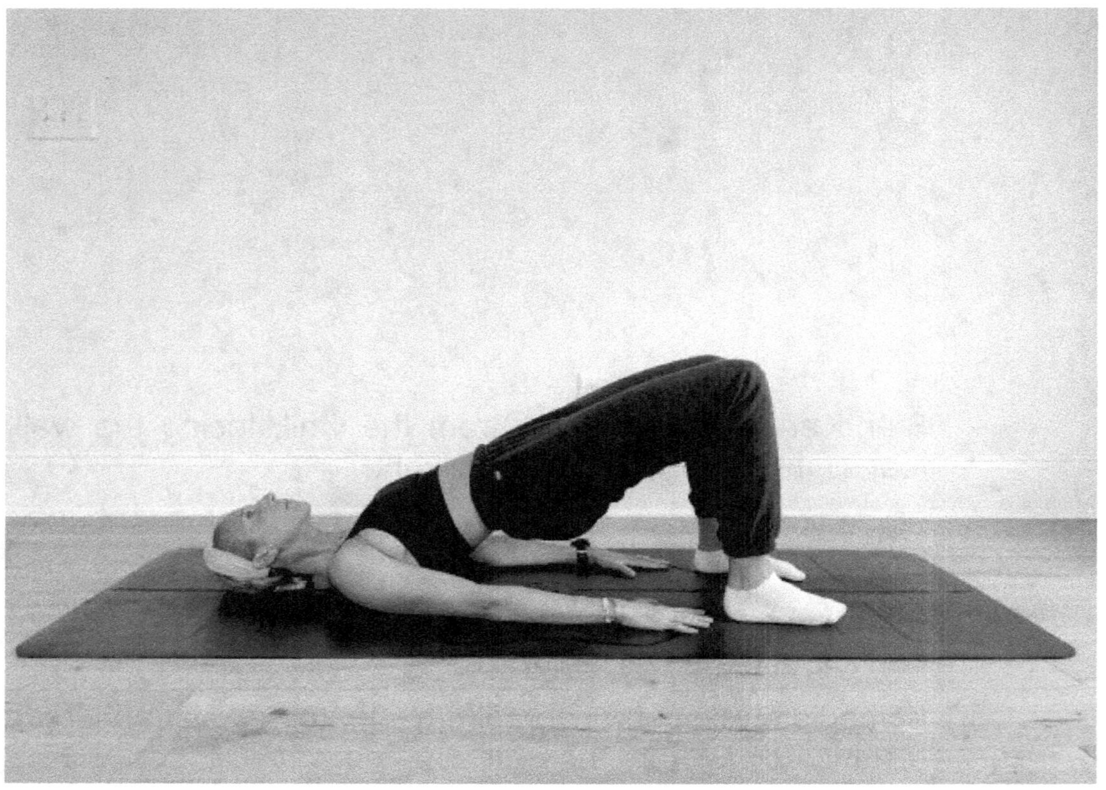

- Lie on your back, on flat, level ground, with your knees bent and feet flat on the ground.

- Your hands should be able to touch the back of your ankles.

- Tighten your abdominal muscles to engage them

- With your glutes, push up into the air. Remain in that position for two seconds.

- Push with your glutes back down to the floor.

- You can include breathing in your glute bridges. Exhale when you push up with the glutes and inhale when you push back down.

- Repeat this ten times without stopping.

#: Side Planks

Planks are modifiable in many ways. The regular front plank may not be very safe after delivery because it causes the abdominal muscles to bulge outwards, which will be the opposite of what we are hoping to achieve. So instead, we opt for a side plank which is a very effective and safe exercise after pregnancy.

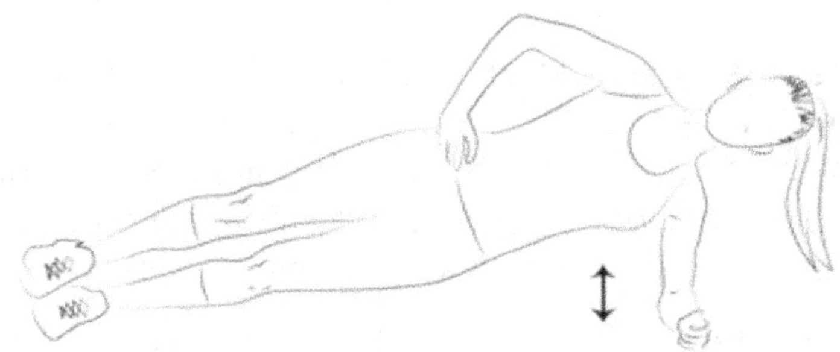

- Lie sideways on flat ground—your elbow on the mat and ensure the elbow aligns with your shoulder. Also, ensure that your hips align with your shoulder so you're neither bending forward nor back.

- Your leg should stretch straight.

- Engage your abdominal muscles, gently raise your hips, then return to the initial position.

- Repeat ten times and then turn to the other side. Repeat the same steps for the other side as well.

If you feel that the above side plank is challenging, you can modify it to have your knees bent instead of stretched out straight.

There is an easier version of the side plank where, instead of supporting yourself with the elbow, you support yourself with the arms.

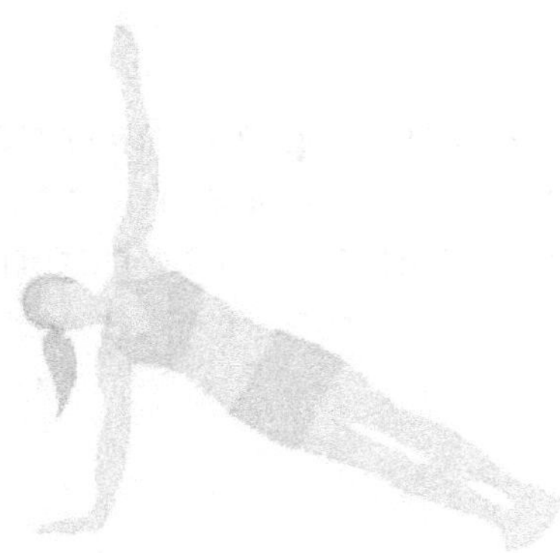

- Can you remember the earlier position when we did a side plank on the elbow? In this exercise, instead of having the elbow on the ground, have your hand on the ground, shoulder and wrist aligned, and find balance by raising the other hand in the air towards the ceiling.

- Have your foot right on top of the foot on the ground or cross your feet to have one in front of the other.

- Hold your hips at the center by engaging the glute and the abdominal muscles. Your hips should not drop too low or go too high. Rather, you should strive to maintain them at the center –that is the challenge.

- Hold that position for 15 to 30 seconds. Take a two-second break and repeat three times.

Another modification of the side planks will be the **Wall planks** which, instead of sitting, you will be standing at arm's length from the wall:

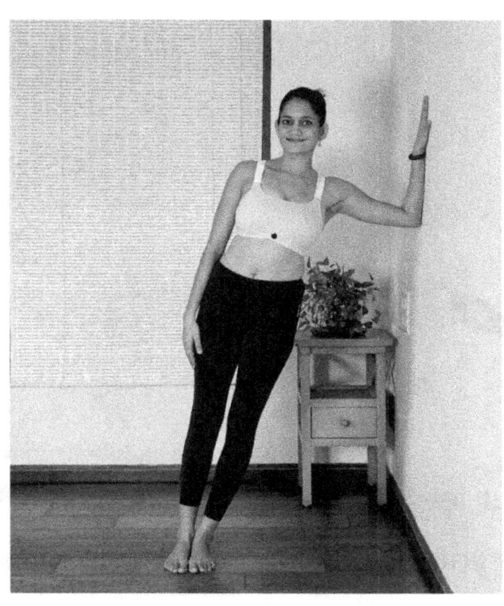

- Stand at stretched arm's length from the wall.

- Position your elbow on the wall so that you are supported against the wall by the elbow –as shown in the image above.

- The pelvis and the spine should be in an aligned position.

- Engage your abdominal muscles by drawing them inside.

- Hold on to this position for 15 to 30 minutes. If you do it correctly, you will begin feeling this exercise working the abdominal muscles on the side next to the wall.

- Repeat these same steps on the other arm for 15 to 30 seconds

- Repeat this exercise three times for each side, giving yourself a break of two seconds

#: Hand walk or Inchworm exercises

The inchworm exercise exercises your core, arms, and shoulders.

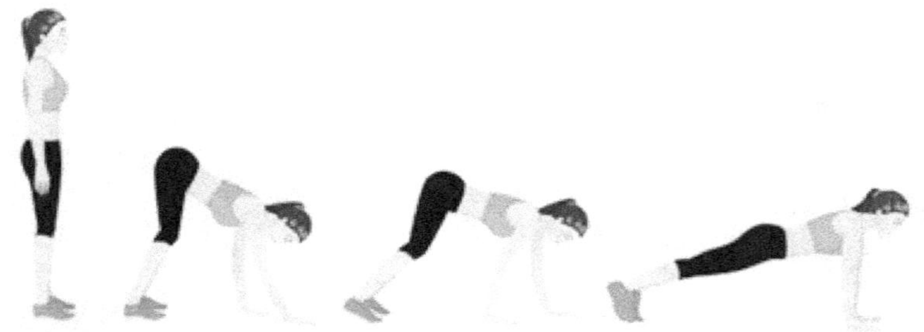

- Stand on flat ground with your feet shoulder length apart.

- Hinged from your hips, place your hand on the ground.

- Begin walking forward with your hands as far as you can.

- When you have reached the furthest point, begin walking backward to return to where you began,

- When you reach your starting point, straighten your legs while still bending, and then stand upright.

- Repeat this ten times. You can give yourself a five-second break, then do another ten walks three times.

To add more intensity, you can do a pushup when you hand-walk to a pushup position, then walk back to the starting point.

#: Hollow body holds

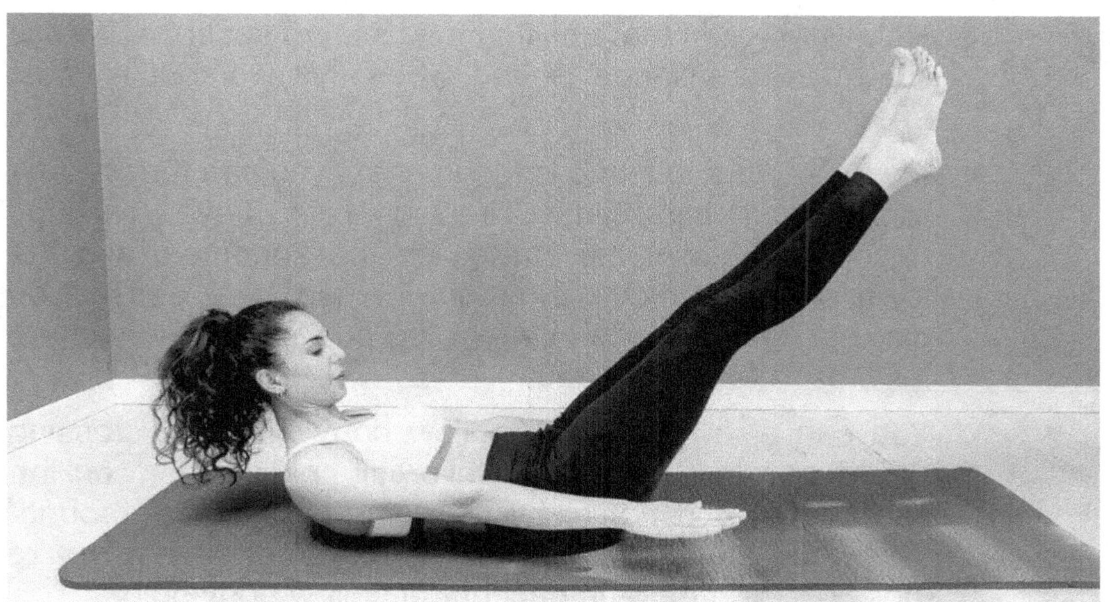

Hollow body holds are basic core exercises. However, they are not as easy as you may have thought, and you are about to find out why.

- Lie on flat ground, with your body against the ground.

- Engage your abdominal muscles by hardening the pelvis and the abdominal muscles. Avoid the abdominal muscles forming a cone because it will make the abdominal muscles bulge outwards even further.

- Lift your knees, pulling them towards your chest.

- Ensure your upper back is pressed to the floor, and slightly lift your head and upper back.

- Place your arms straight against the ground.

- Now stretch out your feet straight, extend them out, and leave them in the air –see the image above.

- Hold yourself in that position for 10 to 15 seconds. That is where the challenge is and when this workout is most effective.

- If you feel that this one is too intense, you can modify it by raising your legs higher. The higher you have your legs raised, the lesser the stretch on the abdomen, and the lower your feet move, the more intense the exercise. You can play around with different leg positions to see where it's most effective for you.

- You can also modify the hollow body holds by crossing your feet interchangeably while still holding them on the same level and not allowing them to touch the ground. This modification is somewhat more intense if you're looking to feel more impact of the hollow body holds.

#: Dead Bug-Bent Legs Only

The dead bug is a core strengthening exercise.   It is one of the friendliest variations of the dead bug exercises.

The regular dead bug exercise that involves movement of your hands and feet is something you should avoid for at least twelve months, especially in the case of diastasis recti, because it causes the abdominal muscles to cone out, causing the abdominal separation to widen.

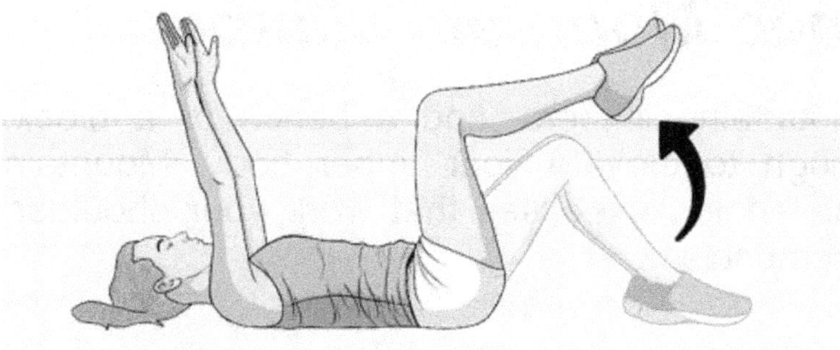

- Lie flat on your back.

- Raise your arms straight in front of you to face the ceiling.

- Bend both your knees and hips to a 90-degree angle.

- Maintain a neutral spine and engage your abdominal muscles.

- Lower one foot in a bent-knee position, controlling it not to touch the ground, then bring it back to the 90-degree position

- Lower the other foot, ensuring you control it not to touch the ground, then bring it back to the 90-degree angle.

- Repeat these moves ten times for each leg.

- Do two sets and take a 10-second break between the sets.

You can alter the leg-only dead bug exercise.

- Instead of lowering your foot in a bent-knee position, extend it straight without touching the ground. Hold it for a few seconds and return it to the 90-degree angle.

- Repeat for the other foot.

- Do the moves ten times for each leg in two sets.

#: Slow Inclined Mountain climber

To do the inclined mountain climbers, find a bench or a block, something stable enough to elevate your upper body. Mountain climbers are good, challenging exercises that work your shoulder, core, triceps, and chest muscles.

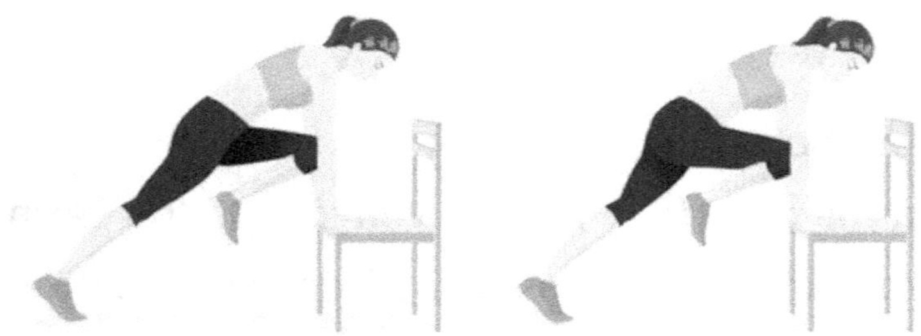

There will be a bit of modification, which sets this inclined mountain climbers from the regular mountain climbers. The regular mountain climbers may not be the best for you at this point. In fact, you should avoid them at all costs because it's hard to control your abdominal muscles from forming a cone, especially with fast movements. That is not to say you should avoid them forever, but give yourself enough time before you can come back to them.

- Assume a pushup position on your bench or block. Ensure your spine is neutral.

- Harden your core to engage it.

- Slowly bring one of your knees towards your chest but not to your chest. If you bring it to your chest, it will be challenging to maintain a neutral spine. Then return to the pushup position.

- Switch up the legs. Bring the other knee towards your chest and return to the pushup position.

- Repeat this ten times for each leg.

- Do three sets of 10 repetitions from each leg, taking a break of ten seconds after each set

If you find this too easy, you can intensify the mountain climber by lowering the height of your inclination or holding your knee longer before returning it to the ground. Something not to forget is that your spine should remain neutral.

#: Bird dog holds

The bird dog holds are good exercises for your abdominals and lower back. They work the spine, abdominal muscles, and glute muscles. These exercises can help you develop and improve your posture when done correctly.

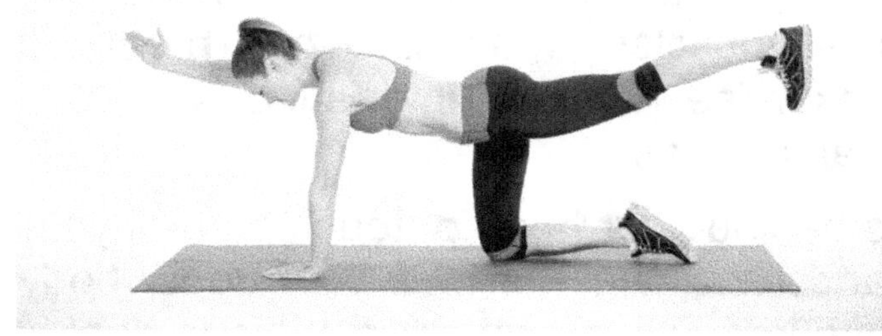

- Start in a quadruped position. Your knees should be in line with your hips and shoulders in line with your wrists.

- Keep your back straight and pull in your abdominal muscle.

- Raise one leg and extend it backward, keeping it straight.

- Extend the opposite arm straight in front of you.

- Hold in that position for 30 seconds.

- Switch up to the other leg and arm and follow the same steps.

- Do three sets of ten repetitions for each side.

- If you'd like to make it more challenging, you can pull your elbow inwards to meet your knee. And repeat three sets of ten repetitions for each leg.

#: *Vacuum twists*

Vacuum twists may seem easy, and they are, but they are also fun and very effective for strengthening your core muscles and slimming your waistline. They are also very effective at repairing the diastasis recti.

- Stand upright with your spine neutral and straight.

- Keep your legs shoulder-length apart.

- Involve your breathing by exhaling, inhaling, then drawing in your abdominal muscles. Maintain your breathing throughout the exercise without interfering with the drawn-in abdominal muscles.

- Place your hands behind your head or touch both of your ears with your hands and begin to twist your upper body from right to left and immediately return from left to right.

- Do five sets of ten repetitions for each side.

There is another version of the vacuum twists that involves using a broomstick.

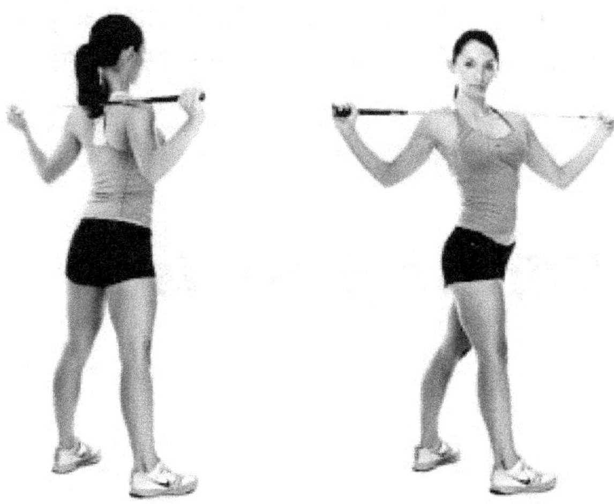

- Stand upright with your spine straight and neutral.

- Your feet should be shoulder length apart.

- Engage your abdominal muscles by drawing them in the whole time during the exercise. Engage your breathing but keep the abdominis drawn in.

- Place a broomstick behind your shoulders and hold each end with your hands —as shown in the image above. The broomstick helps with the side-by-side twists.

- Begin to twist your upper body while holding your broomstick right-to-left, left-to-right.

- Do five sets of ten repetitions for each side.

High-Intensity Abdominal Exercises

The high-intensity abdominal workouts are more advanced core workouts that work the deepest core muscles. Doing these exercises correctly requires you to have developed and built a comfortable level of strength in your core muscles. Ideally, these workouts are for mums whose diastasis recti has already healed, and now you're working to build and maintain core strength.

These exercises include:

#: Wind Shield Wipers Exercise

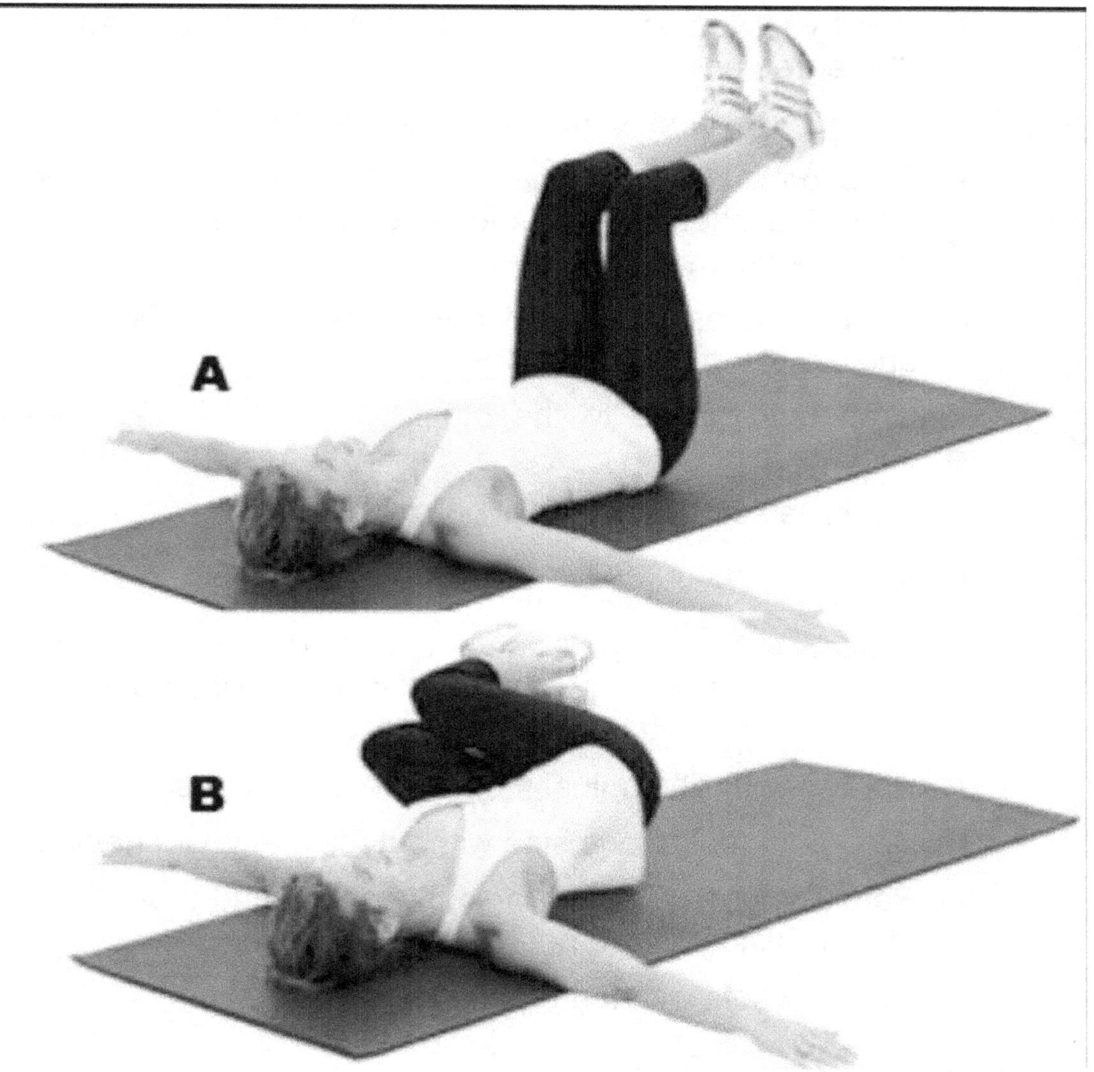

Windshield wipers are great exercises to strengthen the obliques and the rectus abdominis.

- Lie on flat ground, with your spine straight and neutral.
- Spread your arms straight to form a cross.

- Bend your knees to form a 90-degree angle and another 90-degree angle at the hips.

- Harden your abdominal muscles to engage them.

- Drop both knees to one side. Strive to do this without lifting the shoulders off the ground while still hardening your abdominal muscles.

- Lift the knees again and return them to the 90-degree angle.

- Drop both knees to the other side without lifting your shoulders.

- Do three sets of ten repetitions for each side.

If you are ready for a more challenging version of this:

- Instead of having your knees at a 90-degree angle, have your feet straight towards the ceiling, with your spine straight and neutral on the ground.

- Harden your abdominal muscles to engage them.

- Drop both feet to one side without moving your shoulders.

- Return your feet to the original position, and drop them to the other side. Strive not to move your shoulders.

- Do three sets with ten repetitions on both sides.

#: Penguins Taps

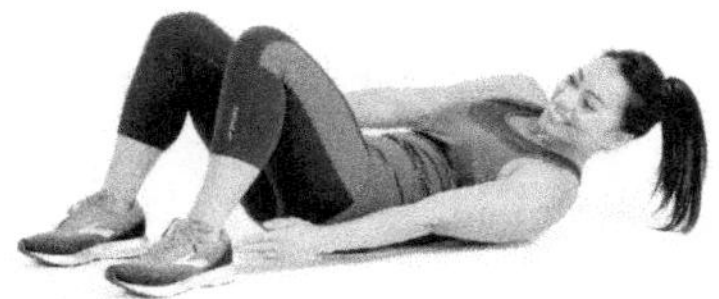

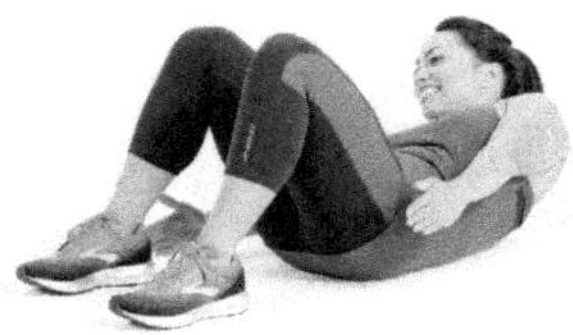

Penguin taps are exercises for your obliques and abdominal muscles. They are named penguins because you make moves like those of a walking penguin.

- Lie flat on the ground, bend your knees, and have your feet straight on the ground.

- Raise your upper back and shoulders.

- The challenge is for your hands to tap the back of your heels.

- Tap the heel on one side with your same side hand, and do the same to the other heel with that other arm.

- These exercises may seem easy, but they are not.

- Do two to three sets of ten repetitions for each side.

#: Standing side crunch

You can do the standing side crunch at a beginner level as well. It targets the oblique abdominal muscle, and after adding some variations, it will work the abdominal rectus muscles as well. Here is how to do it.

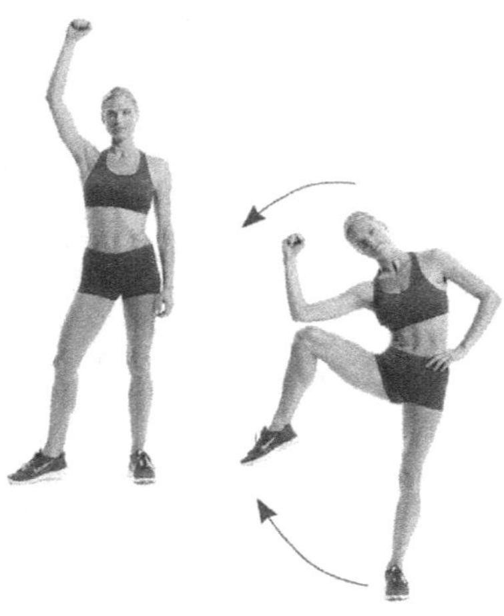

- Stand straight with your feet just slightly apart. Do not bend your spine or knee.

- Place one of your hands on your waist and harden your core.

- Extend the leg on the other side slightly outwards.

- Extend your hand on the same side of the extended leg, from your chest level over your head.

- Lift the knee of the extended leg to touch the elbow of the extended arm. Keep the other leg straight and your hand on the waist. You can either tap the ground every time you lower your foot or touch the ground with your whole foot; either option is fine.

- To add some intensity to the exercise, you can lower your foot to ground level but don't touch the ground. If you must touch the ground, only do it when trying to find balance, and that should happen once in many crunches.

- Repeat this for the other side.

- Do three sets of ten repetitions for each side.

The other variation to this workout adds a twist to the waist by doing a hand-to-knee tap.

- Standing in the same position, place one palm of your hand on the other palm and maintain them at chest level
- Lift the knee of your extended leg to tap it with both your palms. You can make it harder by moving your arms further on the other side so that you will have a deeper twist, almost like you're doing a cross-body crunch or a standing bicycle crunch.
- Do three sets of ten repetitions for each side.

#: *Reverse crunches*

Reverse crunches work your lower abs and are a somewhat challenging exercise that has great rewards. Reverse crunches will be effective even if you don't lift your body too high, as long as you lift your hips correctly.

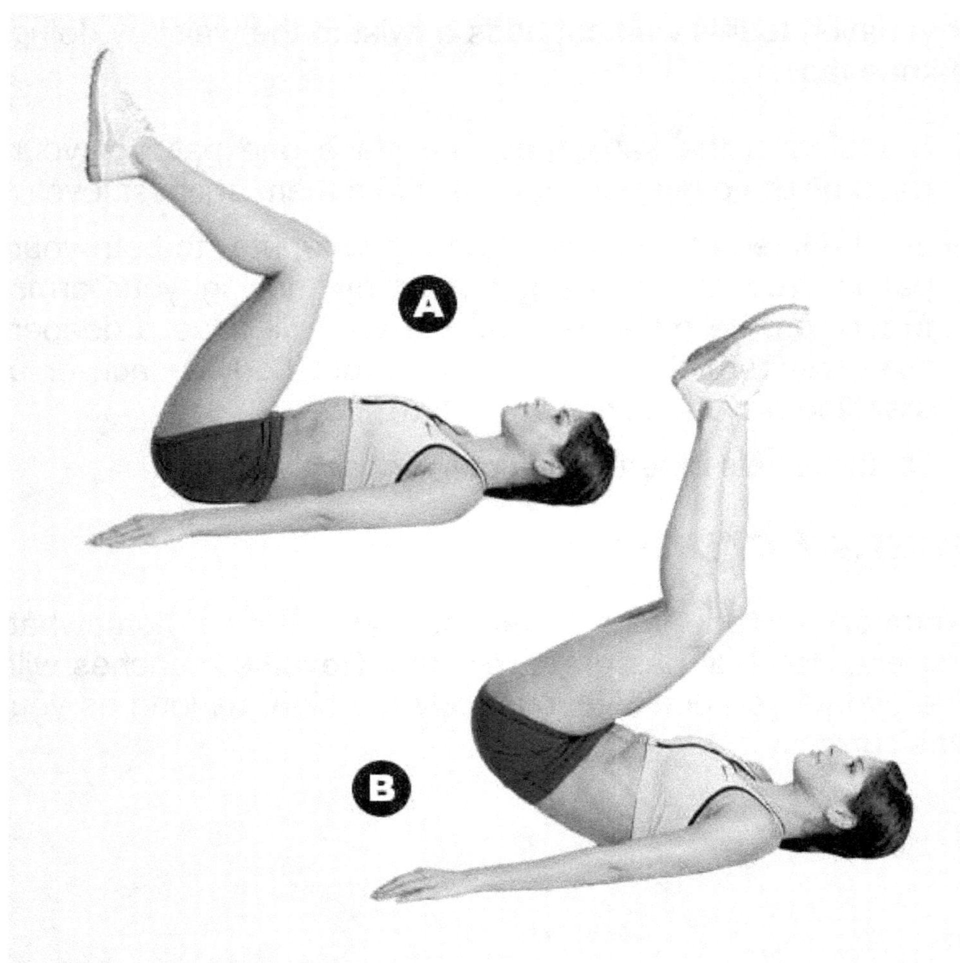

- Lie flat on a flat ground, with your arms on the ground towards your feet, your hips bent 90-degrees, and your knees facing the ceiling but slightly bent as well.

- Harden your abdominal muscles to engage them.

- Raise your hips off the ground and crunch them inwards but do not change the bend on your knees. Try to hold for 2 seconds, then lower your hips to the ground. Also, try not to pull your knees back; rather, lift them upwards.

- Repeat this ten times. You can try to do two sets, taking a break of ten seconds.

To make this a little more challenging,

- Still lying on the ground in the original position, your hips bent 90-degrees, straighten your legs up to the ceiling.

- Place your hands at the back of your head.

- Lift both your head, shoulders, and hips simultaneously.

- Do ten repetitions in two sets.

- If you feel that the modification is too challenging, you have the option to stick to the first one –they both work amazingly well.

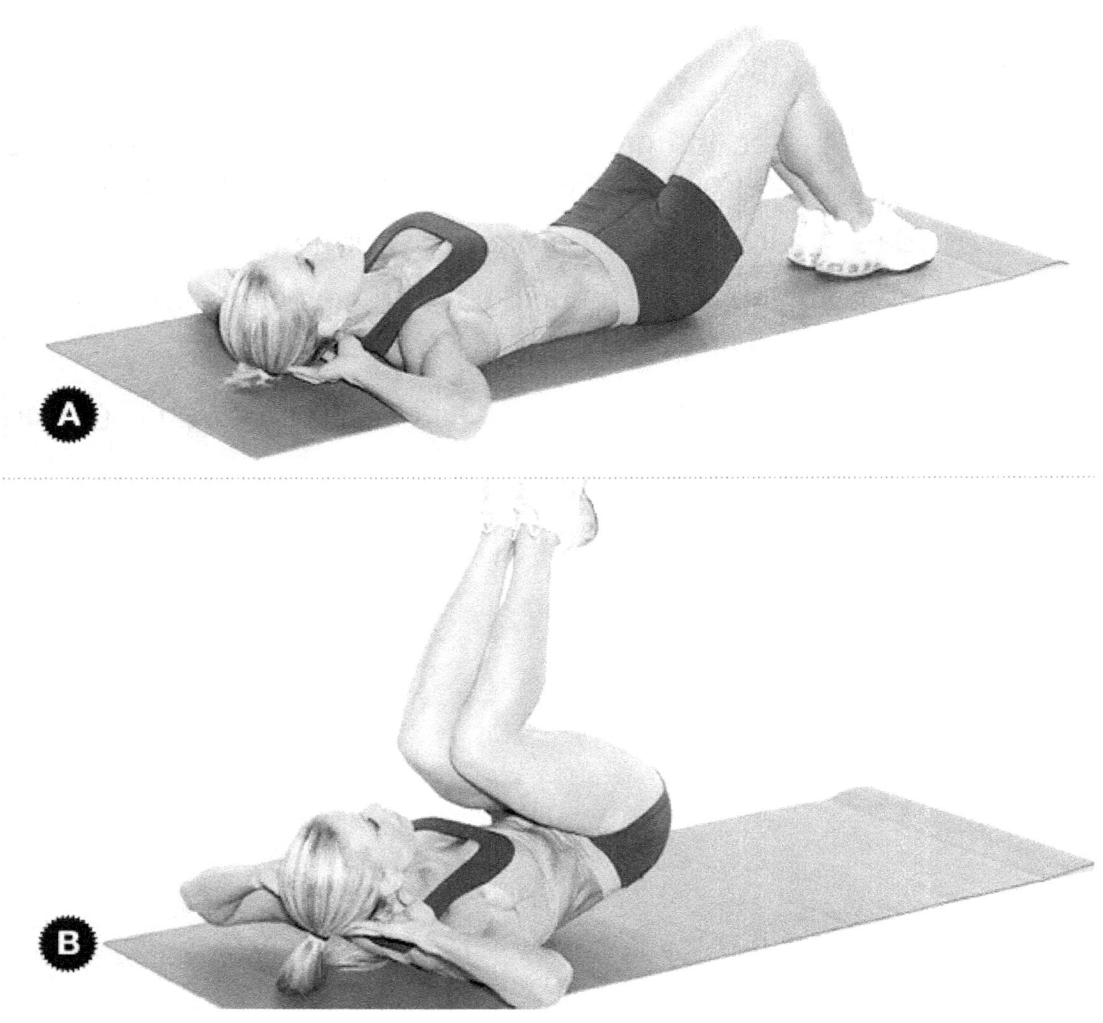

#: Hip Dip Planks

Earlier, you learned how to do the side elbow and wall planks. The hip dip planks are a version of elbow planks, but now you will rotate the hips to work the shoulder, transverse abdominal, oblique, and lower back muscles. The hip dip planks are a bit advanced and need a higher level of core strength.

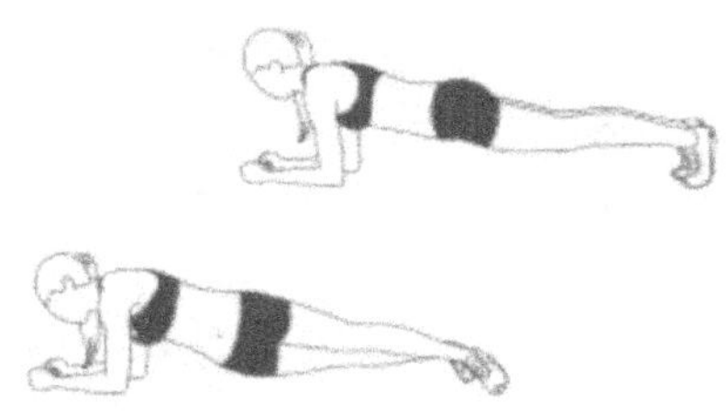

- Lie flat on your stomach on flat ground, with your elbows on the ground and your head lifted, your feet pressing back on your toes.

- Lift your body, hardening your core to engage it. Ensure your spine is straight and neutral to assume a regular plank position.

- In that position, rotate your hips to touch the ground on one side and immediately lift them back to the original plank position.

- Rotate your hips to touch the ground on the other side and immediately return to the original plank position.

- Repeat ten times for each side. Do three sets, giving yourself a break of 10 seconds.

#: Lying Position Bicycle Crunches

The lying position bicycle crunches are similar to the standing bicycle crunches that we looked at earlier. The only difference is that with the lying bicycle crunches, you will be lying on the ground while the standing bicycle crunches are done standing. Also, lying position bicycle crunches are more intense to the core muscles.

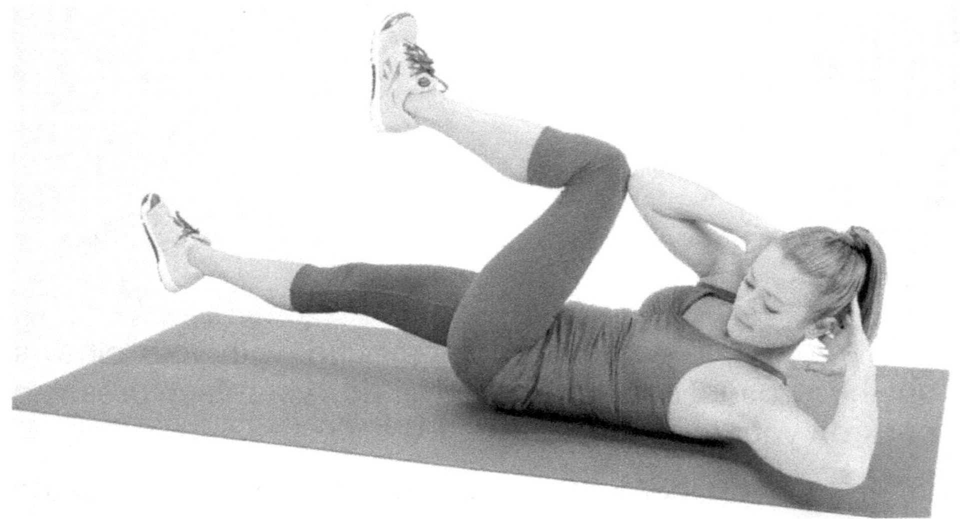

- Lie flat on flat ground with your spine straight and neutral.

- Place your hands at the back of your head. Do not pull your head with your hands, but only place them at the back of your head.

- Lift your legs slightly off the ground

- Harden your abdominal muscles to engage them

- Lift your head and shoulders slightly off the ground as well

- Move your knee towards your chest and your opposite elbow to meet the knee. Do not pull your head with your hands for support when things get hard. That's the wrong way to do bicycle crunches.

- At the same time, extend the other leg outwards. It should not touch the ground at any point.

- Switch up to the other side to repeat the same steps with the other leg.

- Do three sets of ten repetitions for each leg.

#: Flutter Kicks

Flutter kicks will especially work your lower rectus abdominal muscles or what others would call lower abs.

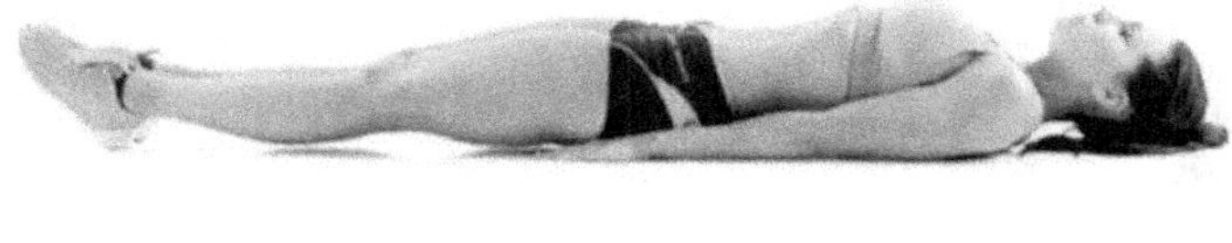

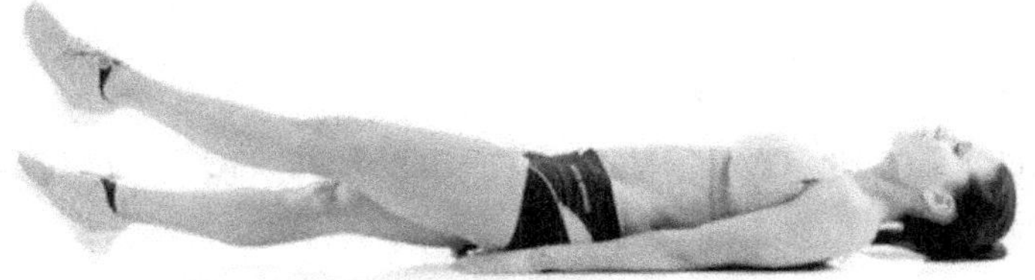

- Lie flat on a flat surface, your head facing the sky and your hands underneath your hips.

- Squeeze and harden your abdominal muscles to engage them.

- Lift both your legs slightly, feet above the ground.

- Lift one leg a little higher, lower it but do not touch the ground, and alternate with the other leg.

- Continue these moves, and do not stop until you have done ten repetitions for each leg.

- To add to the challenge, move your legs faster.

- Do three sets. Take a break of ten seconds after each set.

- If that is still easy for you, add another ten repetitions so that you will be doing twenty repetitions for each leg in one set.

#: The V up Exercise

The V up exercise works both the entire rectus abdominal muscle and the upper and lower rectus abdominal muscle.

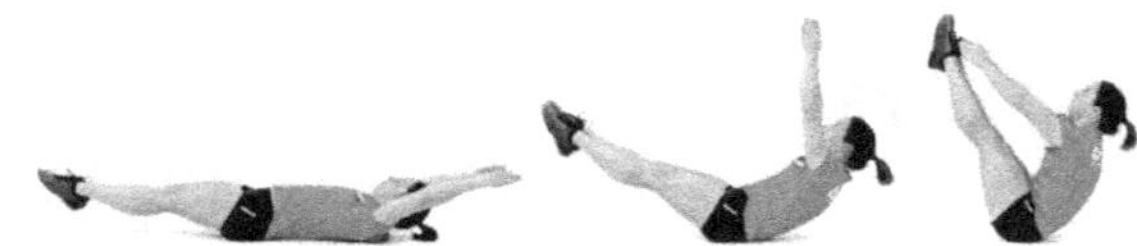

- Lie flat on your back on flat ground.

- Bring both your arms over your head but not to the ground.

- Tighten your abdominal muscles to engage them.

- Keep your legs straight, then lift your legs towards you. With your hands, reach for your toes so that the hands and the toes meet somewhere in the air.

- To make the exercise more challenging, you can hold that position for two to five seconds, then lower your arms and feet.

- Repeat ten times in three sets taking a break of ten seconds each.

#: The Up and Down Plank Exercise

There are endless modifications to planks. The up and down plank is another advanced exercise that is a great challenge to work your abdominal muscles, arms, and shoulder muscles and improve your stability.

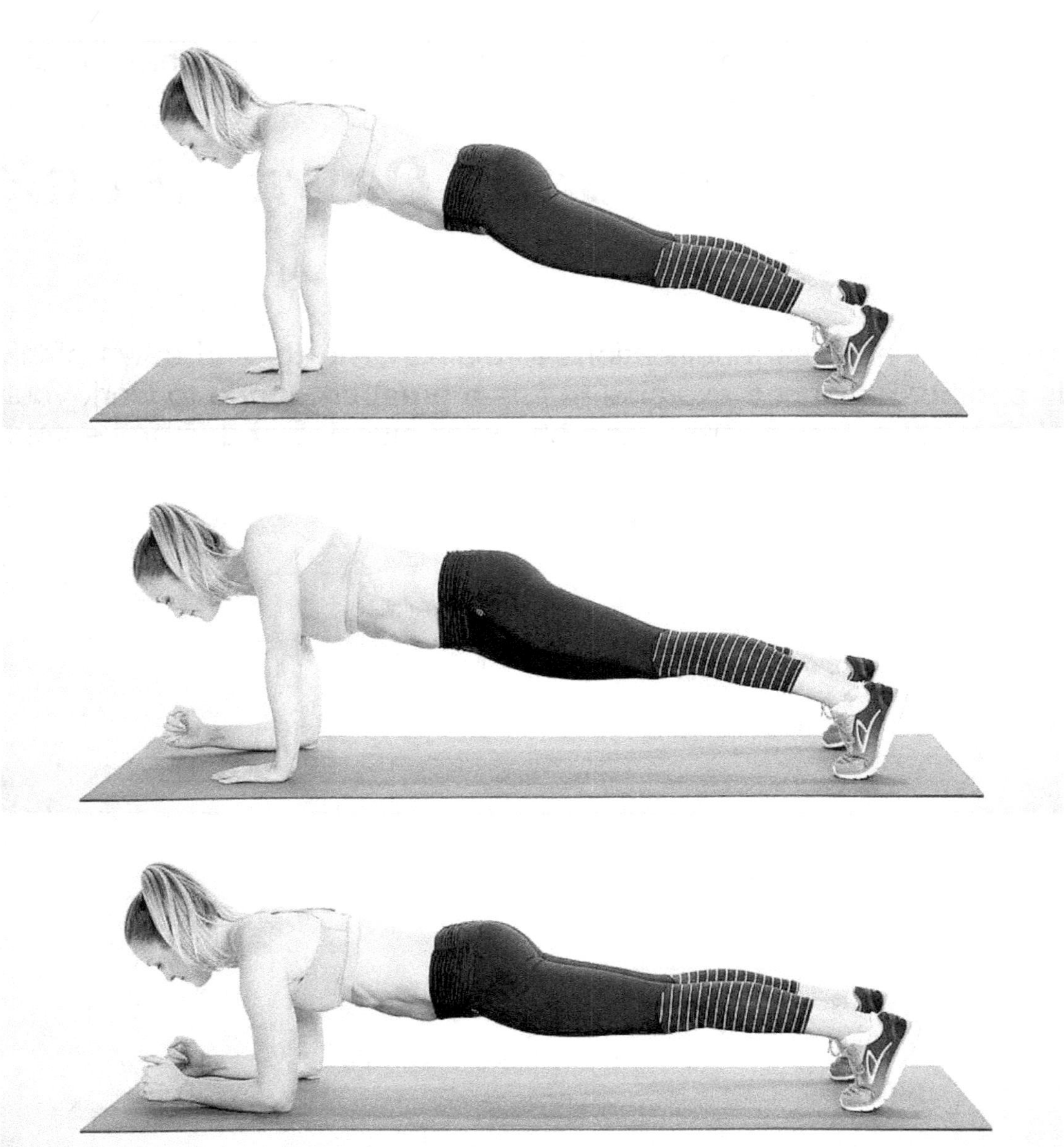

- Assume a pushup position, keeping your back straight, with legs and spine neutral.

- Keep your abdominal muscles tight to engage them.

- Bend your right arm to place your elbow on the ground.

- Bend the other arm to lower yourself to an elbow plank position.

- Raise one arm to straighten it, then the other to return to the pushup position. That is a complete plank.

Repeat ten times for each arm in three sets

#: Roll-up jumps

Roll-up jumps are fun and can also work as cardio workouts that leave you happy with your heart racing while strengthening your core and glute muscles.

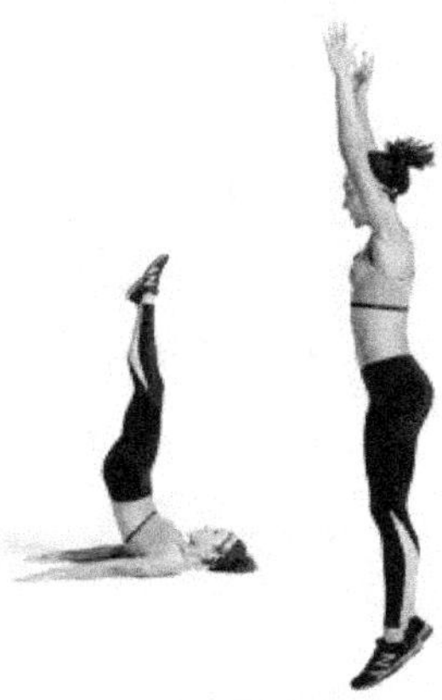

- Sit on flat ground, preferably a soft surface that supports and soothes your back. Bend your knees and have your feet flat on the ground. Your hands apart and behind your butt, fingers facing forward.

- Next, roll back on your back onto your shoulders, lift your hips, and extend your legs towards the ceiling like you're doing a reverse crunch.

- Roll back to the sitting position, but don't sit; use the same momentum to push yourself to your heels and stand up.

- Jump and clap your hands above you, like you would in a burpee. Ensure your back is straight, and do your best to keep your spine neutral as you make the jump.

- Repeat the same moves ten times.

Lower Body/Leg Workouts

Leg workouts, also called glute or lower body workouts, activate your butt, hamstrings, quadriceps, glutes, calves, and even the abdomen —only in some exercises.

Such exercises that are friendly to new mothers include:

#: Air squats

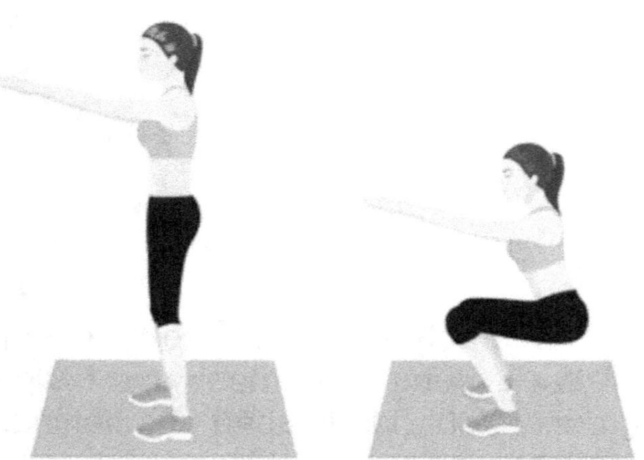

Air squats help your lower body get a good balance and increase blood circulation. When done right, they also improve the health of your joints and target glute muscles, hamstrings, thighs, and quadriceps, and as you try to find balance when squatting, your core gets strengthened.

How to do air squats

- Stand straight on a flat surface. Feet shoulder-width apart, toes slightly turned outwards.

- Move your hips back and downwards, but do not seat.

- Stretch your arms forward in front of you as your butt moves lower.

- Your chest should be nice and flat. You should avoid a situation where you're bending forward.

- Move the hips forwards and stand up; bring your arms to the side facing downwards.

- Ensure that when getting down, your weight is on your heels. Avoid raising your heels; they should be on the ground.

- Your feet should stay slightly turned outwards, and at no point should they be bending inwards. That is the incorrect position.

- Do ten repetitions in five sets, taking a break of five seconds after each set.

#: Side leg raises

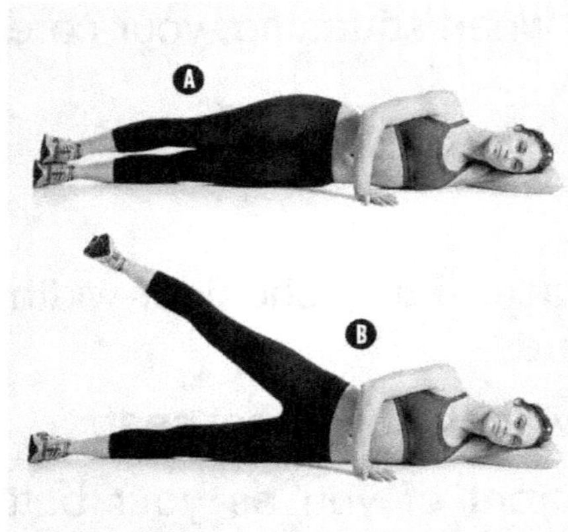

The side leg raises are a glute-strengthening exercise that also strengthens your abdominal muscles, hips, and thighs.

How to do side leg raises

- Lie down on your side on a flat surface.

- As shown in the image above, the lower arm should be under your head, and your upper arm on your hips or can touch the ground.

- Keep your body straight and steady, and engage your abdominal muscles

- Lift your top leg and maintain steady hips and body position. Hold for five seconds, lower it down close to the other leg, then back up.

- Repeat ten times for each leg in five sets.

- To make the leg raises harder, tie something to the ankles of your top leg to make it heavier.

- You can also modify it such that instead of raising your top leg and returning it down, you will raise it and then move it forward while keeping your other leg straight and steady on the ground. You can then take the same leg back behind you and repeat to make a forward and backward swing like movement with your top leg.

- Repeat twenty times for each leg in five sets. A complete leg raise includes the backward and forward swing.

#: Lateral Squat walk

The lateral squat walk is a lower-body strengthening exercise that targets your glutes, inner thighs, and quads. It also strengthens the core since it stays engaged the whole time.

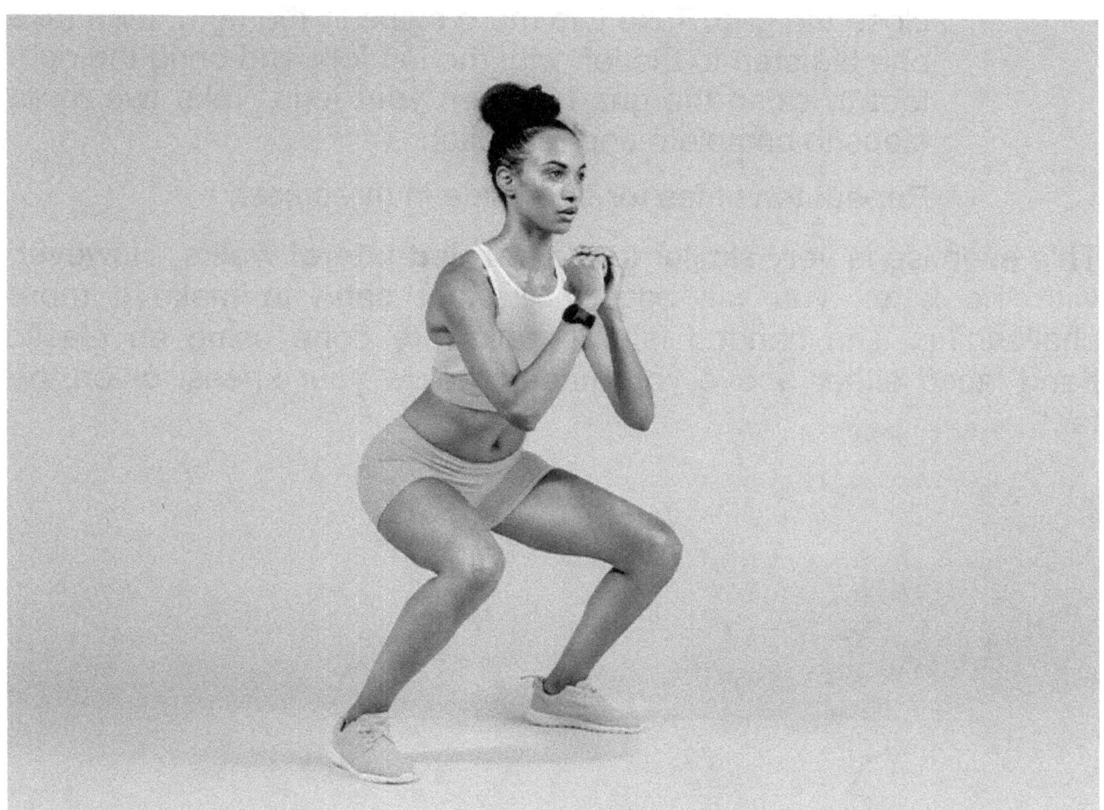

How to do the Lateral Squat walks

- With your legs apart, push your hips behind you and lower them to get into a squat position. Your feet should slightly turn outwards.

- Keep your chest up. Avoid bending forward, but try to maintain an upright upper body posture.

- Tighten your core muscles to engage them. Remember to exhale to tighten the abdominal muscles and then maintain regular breathing.

- In the same squat position, begin by taking a big step to the right with one foot and then bring the other foot to close the gap. Take two more steps to the right, then take one big step to the left with the left foot and bring the right foot to close the gap between your legs. Take two more steps to complete one repetition.

- Repeat ten times for each side in three sets.

This exercise is very similar to the **banded lateral walks**. However, with the latter, you will add a resistant band to make it more challenging. The banded lateral walks are done using an elastic band laced either above your knees, below your knees, or on the feet.

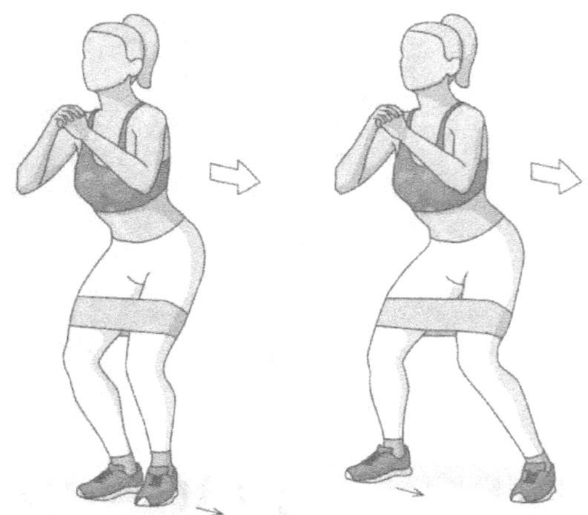

- Place a resistance band above your knees and get into a squat position. Keep the band stretched at all times during the exercise.

- Engage your abdominal muscles and begin by taking a big step to the right with your right foot to create a big stretch on the band. Take a smaller step with the left foot towards your right foot. Taking a smaller step ensures the band will stay stretched. If you close off the gaps between your legs, it will not stretch the band will not be stretched.

- If you have space, take ten steps to the right and ten steps back to the left to complete one repetition. Repeat ten times in three sets.

If you do not have space, you can take three steps to the right, and three steps to the left, then repeat ten times for each side in five sets.

Keep your weight centered and avoid having it on either foot.

#: Squat jumps

Squat jumps or jump squat is one killer workout that is both cardio and lower body workout that targets to race your heart and work those glute, hamstrings, and quad muscles.

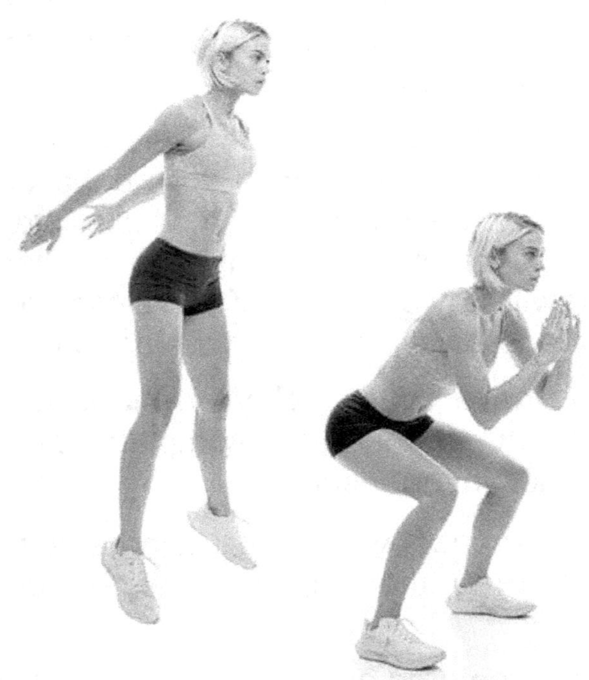

<u>How to do squat jumps</u>

- Start in a squat position, building the tension in the thighs, putting pressure on your butt, and placing your hands together in front of you.

- Pull your hands downwards and jump up and land low on bent knees in the same squat position that you started in

- You should have your chest lifted and the shoulders pulled back.

- Do ten repetitions in three sets.

#: Donkey kicks

Donkey kicks strengthen your glutes and core.

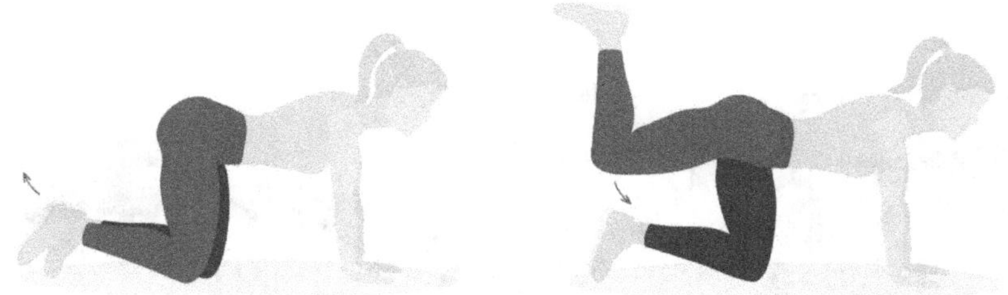

How to do donkey kicks

- Get into a cat position, with your shoulders aligning with your wrists and knees aligned with your hips.

- Engage your abdominal muscles to strengthen the back and core

- Lift your chin and your eyes to look straight ahead.

- Squeeze your glutes and lift your right leg behind you towards the ceiling. The left leg should be in the same cat position, and your back should be neutral.

- Lift your leg to slightly above your butt and bring it down to the floor but don't touch the floor, immediately lift it again and keep going until you have completed ten repetitions.

- Do three sets of ten repetitions for each leg.

Do not rush so that you will maintain the proper posture.

The donkey kicks are very similar to the mini band kickbacks

With the miniband kickbacks, you will use an elastic band that can be improvised with anything elastic and stable at home.

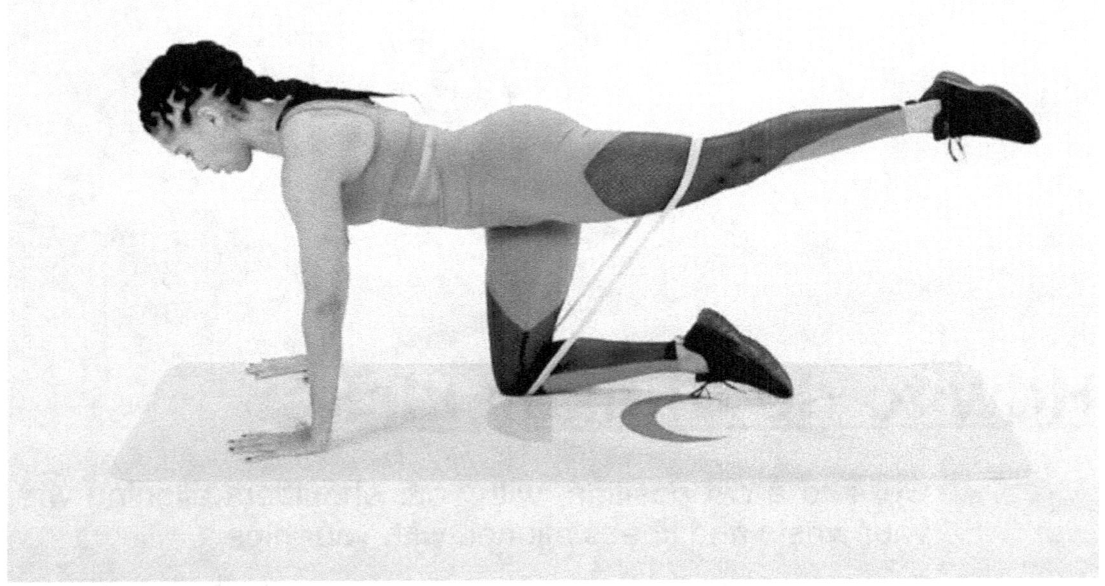

How to do the miniband kickbacks

- Start in a cat position with your shoulders aligned with your wrist, hips aligned with your knees, and spine neutral and stable.

- Place a mini elastic band around your right foot and the other end above the left knee. The elastic band should be stretched between your right foot and left knee.

- Keep your abdominal muscles tight and glutes squeezed.

- Extend your right foot back until it's fully straight, then bring it back.

- Repeat ten times for each leg in three sets.

#: Marching Glute bridges

Earlier, we looked at how to do the glute bridges as a core workout. You might have noticed by now that most lower body workouts also strengthen the core in the process. The same is true with the marching glute bridges that target the glutes, hamstrings, core muscles and lower back muscles.

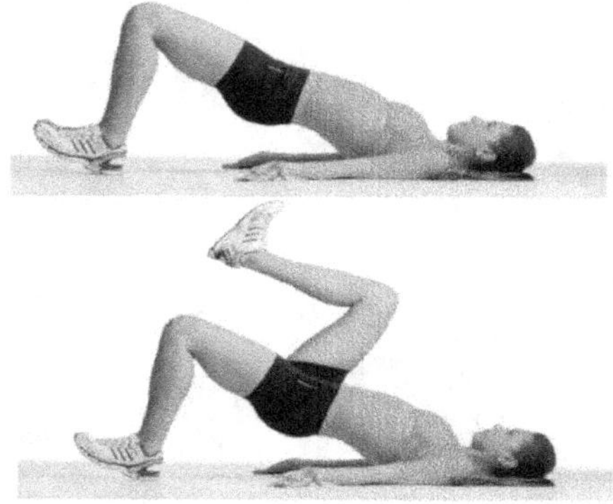

How to do the marching glute bridges

- Lie flat on a flat surface, with knees bent. Ankles should be close to your glute but shouldn't touch it.

- Squeeze your glutes and engage your abdominal muscles for full results.

- Lift your hip, and ensure that your back is neutral and stable enough. That will bring you to a glute bridge position.

- Lift your right foot off the ground, push it towards you, then bring it back to the start glute bride position. Lift the left foot using the same steps. That is one repetition.

- Do ten repetitions for each leg in three sets.

#: *Reverse lunges*

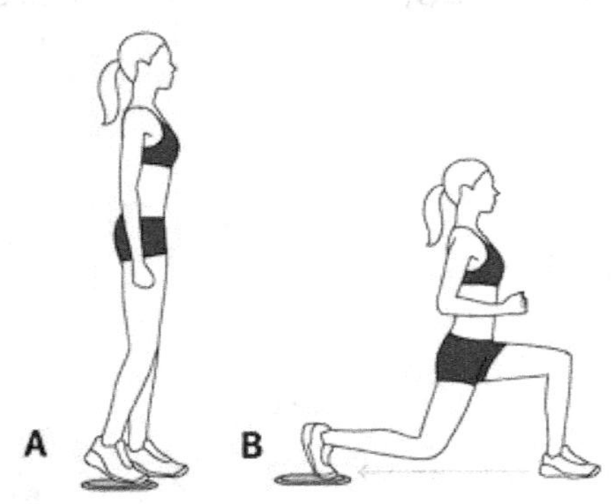

Reverse lunges are stability workouts that activate your core, glutes, and hamstrings.

How to do reverse lunges

- Start in a standing position on a flat surface.

- Step your right leg back and kneel the knee while maintaining an uplifted chest position. Hold for three seconds and come back up.

- If you have weights, you can hold a dumbbell on the side of the bending knee.

- Do ten repetitions for each leg in three sets.

#: Lunge skips

The lunge skip is another challenging yet refreshing and effective lower body workout that strengthens the glutes and core and raises your heartbeat.

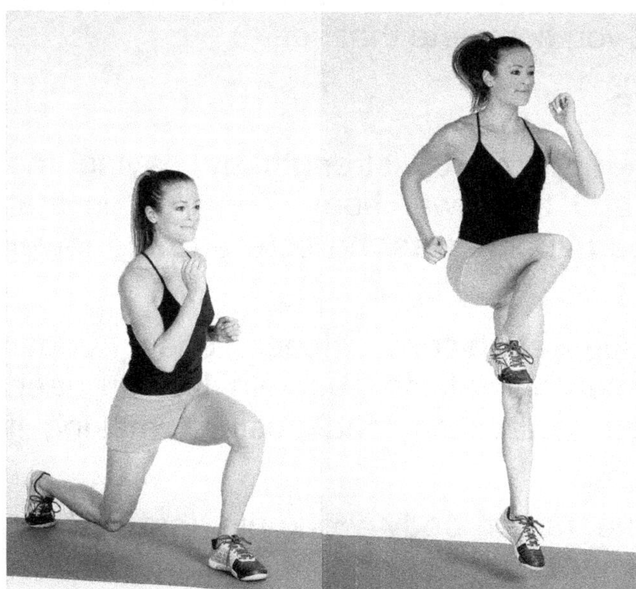

How to do lunge skips

- Stand straight on flat ground.

- Engage your abdominal muscles and step back with your right foot, lowering your knee close to the ground but not touching the ground.

- The left foot hinges to a 90-degree angle at the hips and knee.

- Bring the right knee forward and up towards your chest and make a jump as your right knee goes up.

- Repeat this move ten times on both legs in three sets.

- Ensure to keep your spine neutral and stable.

- You can modify this if you're not comfortable skipping so that instead of jumping when your knee is moving towards your chest, you will bring your knee towards your chest and return it to the lunge position without moving your other leg until you complete that set.

Upper Body Workouts

Many people often overlook upper body strength by paying too much attention to the belly and the lower body. The truth is that upper body strength is just as important as the core and the lower body strengths.

Upper body strength encompasses biceps, triceps, chest, upper back, shoulders, neck, and even part of the abdominals. You need upper body strength for good metabolism and posture, making it easier to run your daily errands.

Some incredible and effective upper body workouts that will do wonders for your everyday life include.

#: Inclined pushups

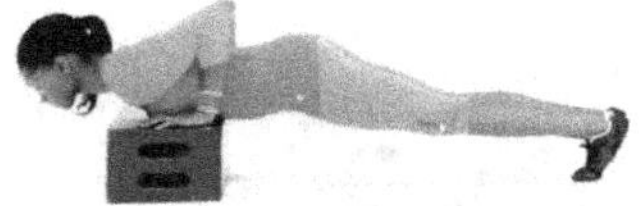

The inclined pushup is a modified pushup that works your chest and core.

How to do the inclined pushups

- Start in a plank position with your hands on a bench or a box and feet straight behind you.

- Your back should be straight and neutral, palms on the bench facing forward, chest straight, and shoulders neutral.

- Ensure to engage your abdominal muscles to help protect your back.

- Bend your arms slowly as you lower your chest towards the bench or box, then slowly straighten your arms to lift your chest back to the plank position.

- Repeat ten times in three sets. You can increase the number of sets as you get stronger.

The traditional pushup is also an excellent upper body workout that strengthens your shoulders, chest, and arms. It challenges many women initially, but as you build your upper body strength, you will notice that it will become much easier.

How to do pushups

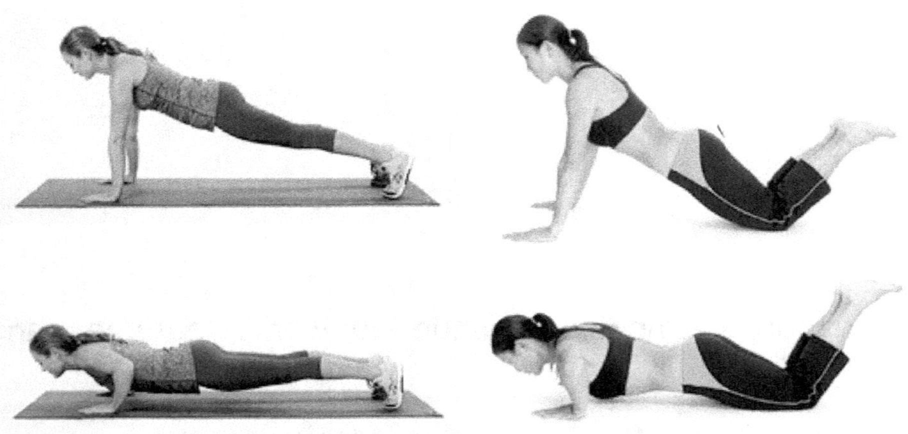

- Start in a plank position, hands on the ground, fingertips facing forward.

- Ensure to keep your back neutral and hands shoulder-width apart to avoid injuries and incorrect posture. Also, engage your core muscles to protect your back.

- Lower your arms to lower your body to the ground up to a point where your back will be straight, and then straighten your arms to bring yourself back up to a plank position.

- Repeat ten times in three sets, and you can do this daily.

#: Plank shoulder taps

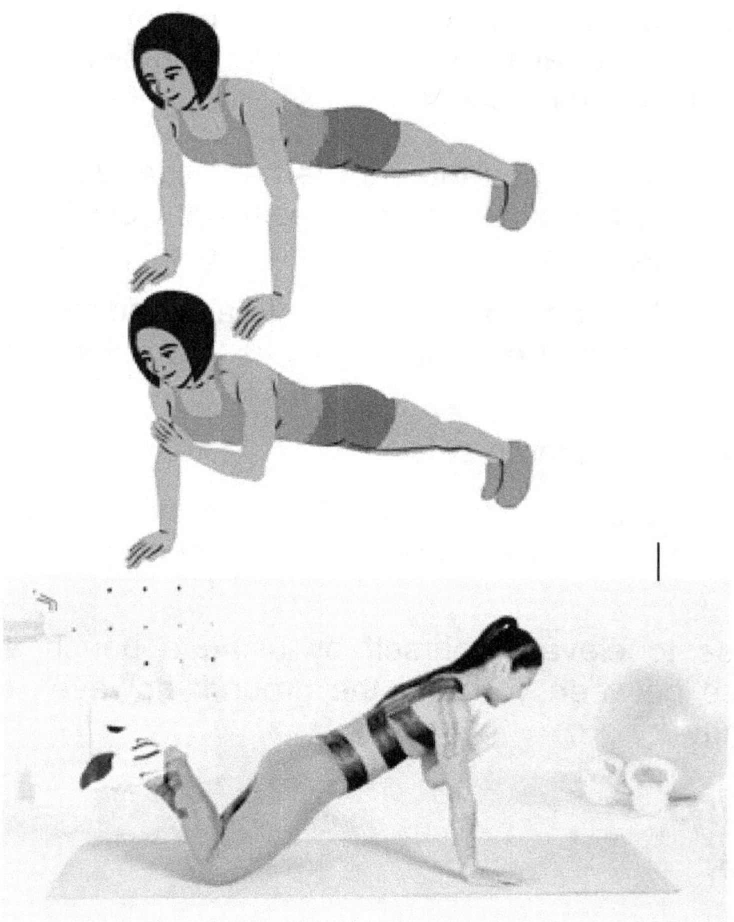

The plank shoulder taps are very efficient workouts for shoulders, arms, and core because doing them engages and strengthens all these muscles.

How to do the shoulder planks

- Start in a plank position, back neutral, your core engaged, hands on the ground and fingertips facing forward, shoulders neutral to avoid having a wrong posture.

- You can choose to have your knees on the ground and interlock your feet behind you if you find it easier. Either way, you get the same results.

- Take your right palm and tap your left shoulder while the rest of the body remains in a plank position. Hold for two seconds and return the right arm to the original position.

- Alternate hands and then take your left palm and tap your right shoulder using the same moves as you did with the right hand.

- Repeat ten times in three sets.

There are variations to the shoulder taps. We already mentioned one of them where you bend your knees and interlock your feet behind you.

You can also choose to elevate yourself by using a bench and reducing the distance between you and the ground; however, the moves remain the same.

#: Triceps dip

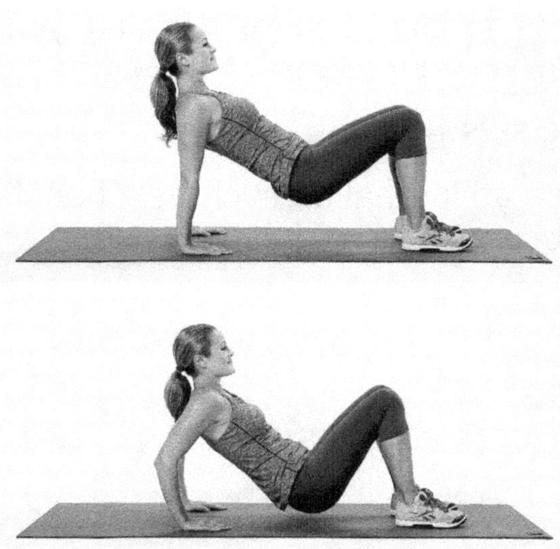

Tricep dips are a total body exercise that works to build your shoulders and arms strength.

How to do tricep dips

- Sit down on a flat surface, with your leg stretched out and your back straight, forming an L shape from your hips.

- Bend your knees in so that they will provide support, and place your hands behind your hips, making sure your arms are not too far from your body —your fingertips should point towards you.

- Bend your arms slightly and lift your hips off the floor. Lift your hips, then slowly straighten your arms to support your body while in the lifted hips position.

- Ensure your neck is straight, your shoulders neutral, and your elbows under your shoulders; they should be straight and not wide apart.

- Slowly drop your hips off to the ground, bending your arms and putting pressure on your triceps.

- Repeat ten times in three sets.

To modify the tricep dip, you can use an inclination such as a bench, chair, or another evenly raised surface.

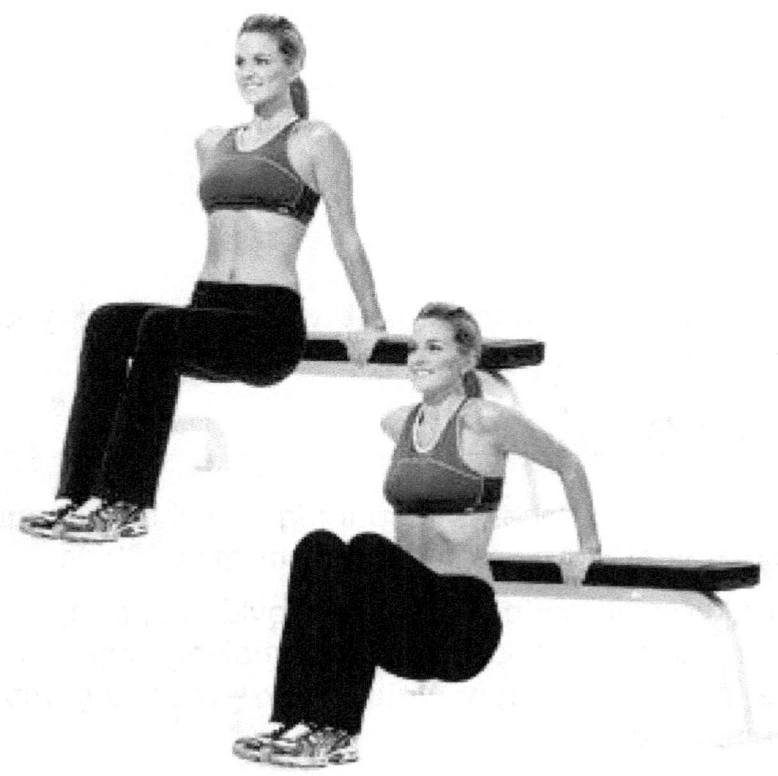

- Sit on the bench with your hands beside your hips, with your fingertips holding the bench and facing forward. Keep the knees bent in front of you.

- Move your hips off the bench and have it just against it; your hands should be supporting you at this point.

- Lower your hips against the bench until your arms are parallel to the floor, then lift your hips back to the bench level but do not seat.

- Repeat ten times in two sets.

#: *Resistance band pull-apart*

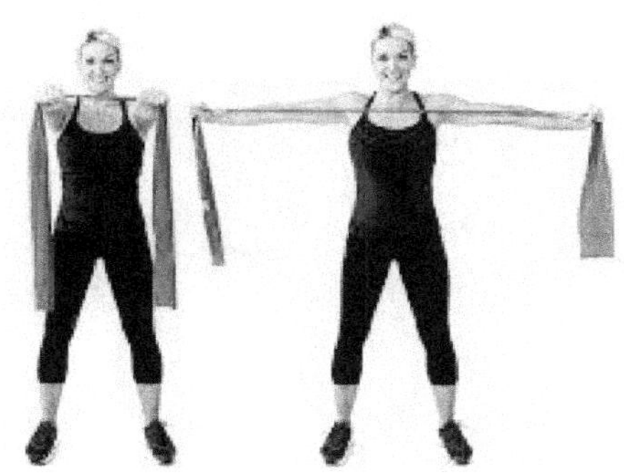

Resistant band pull-apart is a simple exercise that will work your upper back muscles and shoulders. You will need a resistant band, or you can use an elastic fabric or rubber, but carefully to not harm yourself.

How to do the resistant band pull-aparts

- Start by standing on a flat surface with your legs shoulder-width apart, and arms stretched out straight in front of you at chest level while holding the resistant band with your hands, as shown in the above image.

- Engage your core, and ensure you have an upright posture; your face should be up and facing forward.

- Spread both arms straight to form a cross while pulling the resistant band.

- Pull your arms back to the starting position, and repeat.

- Repeat ten times in two sets.

#: Wall Angels

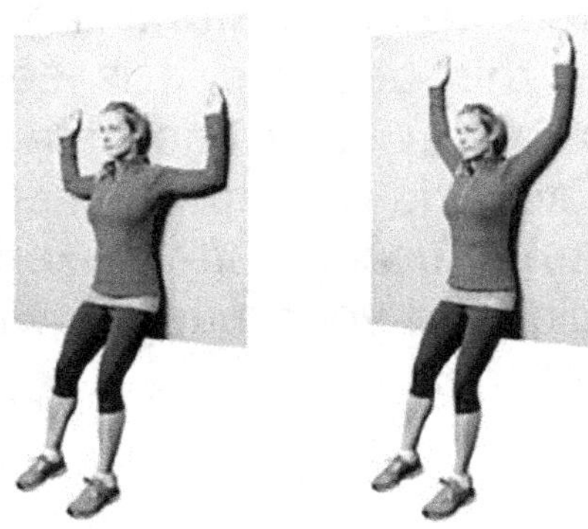

The wall angels seem easy, but you will begin to feel them because you keep your hands lifted.

- Start by standing at the wall, feet about three inches away from the wall

- Lean your hips and back on the wall, shoulders, your back, and back of your arms on the wall.

- Bend your elbow so that your fingertips are facing the ceiling and the back of your palms is against the wall.

- Lift your arms against the wall above your head, bring them back to the level of your head, and repeat.

- Repeat ten times in three sets.

You might have gotten a headache or come across people who have migraines during exercise. That could have been caused by skipping warm-ups. That's why it is always good to start all your workouts by warming up.

When you warm up before exercise, you increase blood and oxygen circulation to your muscles, making your muscles more active and flexible as you exercise. You also prepare yourself mentally and physically.

You might also have noticed that trainers insist on stretching after every workout session. They insist on this because it is equally important to stretch to relax the muscles you have been straining during exercise. The body produces lactic acid during the exercise, which contributes to sore and painful muscles after exercise. Stretching will help reduce the lactic acid, and your muscles will be less painful, increase flexibility and add to the tone.

Chapter 6: Nutrition While Breastfeeding and Exercising

Now you know all the amazing workouts you can do to tone your body and stay energized and confident. Let's talk nutrition.

Nutrition is as important as exercising because it affects your body's energy levels. It is therefore essential that you take care of both.

As a new mother who's breastfeeding, you will require extra calories to cater to your nutritional needs because you're passing on these calories to your baby. You need at least 300 to 400 extra calories. The exact calorie intake will depend on your age, height, sex, and body mass index. A dietitian can help you determine your exact calorie intake

The quality of the food on your plate affects both you and the baby. Therefore, it is crucial to balance your diet for every meal you consume. Some foods come in high quantities and lots of calories, but their quality in terms of the amounts of nutrients they add to the body is lacking. Examples of such foods are junk foods such as chips and desserts. You can eat these once in a while and very controlled potions, but it's not advisable to fill your body with such foods.

Doctors recommend that you do not skip breakfast and have small meals spaced within 2 or 3 hours so you can have around five t0 six meals, and between meals, have some snacks that contain fiber and proteins.

Some healthy foods you can eat to lose weight and keep you –and the baby– energized and healthy include.

- **Drinks:** Water will keep you hydrated and your joints well lubricated, especially during exercise. Fruit juice and milk are also healthy drinks to have. Drinks containing caffeine, like tea, coffee, chocolate, and soda, are best avoided or consumed in minimal quantities. Caffeine is a stimulant that may pass on to the baby –through breast milk–altering the baby's growth. Sweetened beverages are good but may not be very helpful when you're working to shed extra weight.

- **Grains:** These include oats, wheat bread, brown rice, pasta, and cereals. Grains are good for breakfast or any meal of the day. The grains help increase milk supply and provide vitamin B, iron, fiber, and energy to your body.

- **Fruits and vegetables are especially good for vegetarians:** You need to choose ones rich in iron, protein, vitamins, and calcium, such as lentils, greens, cereals, and peas. Some fruits are rich in fiber, and fiber will prevent constipation and help with your metabolism. Consider fruits like oranges, grapes, broccoli, and strawberries for vitamin C. Sweet potatoes, broccoli, carrots, and greens are good sources of vitamin A.

- **Daily products:** Dairy is rich in protein and calcium and includes milk, yogurt, and cheese. Four glasses of milk a day will be a good amount to keep your bones strong and help develop the baby's bones.

- **Meat and cereals:** These are good sources of iron and proteins. Such foods include fish, chicken, beef, pork, nuts, and beans. Eggs can also fall into this category. Protein foods are a good source of energy for your body. It is encouraged that you have proteins in each of your meals.

- **Supplements:** Your doctor may recommend supplements such as B12 and vitamin D. You can easily get this through your diet if you take the right nutrients. Do not take the supplements unless advised by a doctor to avoid excess of any nutrient which may cause other problems to you and the child.

When breastfeeding, you need to avoid certain foods and drinks like a plague.

- Any drinks with even the tiniest percentage of alcohol are harmful to your body. Wine, liquor, beer, and other alcoholic drinks will harm your baby's brain and body development.

- Caffeine is a stimulant that's not good for the baby's body. Although some doctors say it is okay to consume it in minimal amounts, avoiding it all together keeps you and your baby on the safe and healthy side.

- Certain types of fish have contaminants called mercury, which is harmful to the baby's brain and nervous system development –these fish include shark, swordfish, mackerel, and tilefish. Healthy fish include salmon, light tuna, shellfish, tilapia, lobster, sardines, shrimp, and crab.

Besides the foods and drinks you should avoid, most other foods are safe for the baby. You can experiment with your baby's tastes and reactions to different foods to help you choose your diet based on the foods that agree with them.

Conclusion

In conclusion, be realistic about your journey. You should not expect to look like a Hollywood model within a month. You can, but the chances are high that you won't, and that is fine.

Realize that it is a journey, a process that needs discipline and consistency in your diet and exercise. Above all, trust the process, have fun, and sooner or later, you will see the results you want.

PS: I'd like your feedback. If you are happy with this book, please leave a review on Amazon.

Please leave a review for this book on Amazon